YOUR KNOWLEDGE HAS VALUE

- We will publish your bachelor's and master's thesis, essays and papers

- Your own eBook and book - sold worldwide in all relevant shops

- Earn money with each sale

Upload your text at www.GRIN.com and publish for free

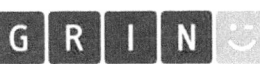

Bibliographic information published by the German National Library:

The German National Library lists this publication in the National Bibliography;
detailed bibliographic data are available on the Internet at http://dnb.dnb.de .

Imprint:

Copyright © 2016 GRIN Verlag, Open Publishing GmbH
Print and binding: Books on Demand GmbH, Norderstedt Germany
ISBN: 9783668311763

This book at GRIN:

http://www.grin.com/en/e-book/341113/the-effects-of-localized-vibration-on-
delayed-onset-muscle-soreness-following

Dr. Fredrick Peters

The effects of localized vibration on delayed onset muscle soreness following intense eccentric cycling

GRIN Publishing

GRIN - Your knowledge has value

Since its foundation in 1998, GRIN has specialized in publishing academic texts by students, college teachers and other academics as e-book and printed book. The website www.grin.com is an ideal platform for presenting term papers, final papers, scientific essays, dissertations and specialist books.

Visit us on the internet:

http://www.grin.com/

http://www.facebook.com/grincom

http://www.twitter.com/grin_com

THE EFFECTS OF LOCALIZED VIBRATION
ON DELAYED ONSET MUSCLE SORENESS
FOLLOWING INTENSE ECCENTRIC CYCLING

A dissertation submitted to the
Kent State University College and Graduate School
of Education, Health, and Human Services
in partial fulfillment of the requirements
for the degree of Doctor of Philosophy

by

Fredrick J. Peters Jr.

May 2016

A dissertation written by

Fredrick J. Peters Jr.

B.A., John Carroll University, 2007

M.B.A., Western Governors University, 2011

Ph.D., Kent State University, 2016

Approved by

_____, Co-Director, Doctoral Dissertation Committee
Angela L. Ridgel

_____, Co-Director, Doctoral Dissertation Committee
J. Derek Kingsley

_____, Member, Doctoral Dissertation Committee
John McDaniel

_____, Member, Doctoral Dissertation Committee
Ellen Glickman

_____, Member, Doctoral Dissertation Committee
Lisa Chinn

Accepted by

_____, Director, School of Health Sciences
Lynne E. Rowan

_____, Interim Dean, College of Education, Health and
Mark Kretovics   Human Services

PETERS JR., FREDRICK J., Ph.D., May 2016   HEALTH SCIENCES

THE EFFECTS OF LOCALIZED VIBRATION ON DELAYED ONSET MUSCLE
SORENESS FOLLOWING INTENSE ECCENTRIC CYCLING (106 pp.)

Directors of Dissertation: Angela L. Ridgel, Ph.D.
                             J. Derek Kingsley, Ph.D.

Delayed onset muscle soreness (DOMS) is musculoskeletal pain resulting from

physical activity. DOMS affects athletic performance, therefore therapy is of interest to

athletes. The purpose of this study was to examine the effects of localized vibration

(biomechanical muscle stimulation, BMS) on biomarkers of DOMS following eccentric

cycling, and to test changes in muscle length and soreness. We investigated if BMS

reduces DOMS and enhances muscle function following eccentric exercise and if creatine

kinase (CK), lactate, and pain were affected. Twenty-eight recreationally active men (18

– 40 years old) were randomized into control or BMS groups. Subjects performed 5

minutes of eccentric cycling, then either received BMS, or rested. Outcome variables,

plasma creatine kinase, blood lactate, pain scores (Likert), muscle length, muscle pain

(self-reported), and pressure algometry were collected at four intervals (baseline,

pre-cycling, 24 hours post-cycling, and 48 hours post). A main effect of time was found

for quadriceps pain threshold ($F(3, 78) = 3.02, p = 0.04$). A main effect of time was

found regarding an increase in lactate ($p = .016$; T0 to T1) and decrease in lactate ($p

= .025$; T1 to T3). A main effect of time for Likert pain score was found pre-cycling

versus post-cycling ($p = .0001$). There were no significant interactions between group

(BMS or control) and time. This study does not support our hypotheses regarding localized vibration and recovery from DOMS. However, we found significance regarding a main effect of time for pain threshold in the quadriceps, Likert pain score, and lactate level.

TABLE OF CONTENTS

LIST OF FIGURES

LIST OF TABLES

CHAPTER I

INTRODUCTION

Following unaccustomed physical activity, a sensation of discomfort occurs in the skeletal muscle known as delayed onset muscle soreness (DOMS) (Cheung, Hume, & Maxwell, 2003). DOMS can adversely affect muscular performance due to voluntary reduction of effort and from inherent loss of capacity of the muscles to produce force (Armstrong, 1984). DOMS is induced by unfamiliar or excessive exercise that temporally produces metabolites and by-products of tissue damage in the body. Furthermore, DOMS results in inefficient blood supply and lack of oxygen in the contracting muscle, leading to pain, muscle weakness, decline of muscle length, and reduction of proprioceptive ability (Cheung et al., 2003).

Theodore Hough first provided a description of DOMS in 1902 as "a kind of soreness that is fundamentally the result of ruptures within the muscle" (Hough, 1902). Eccentric exercises, such as downhill running, eccentric cycling, and resistance training are other common methods for inducing DOMS. Eccentric contractions initiate a cascade of inflammatory responses (Baird, Graham, Baker, & Bickerstaff, 2012). This process of muscle injury and disruption is not entirely understood; though it is thought to consist of a series of events involving oxidative stress, inflammation and immune responses (Baird et al., 2012). Researchers have shown that the type of force development during eccentric exercise may cause disruption of the sarcomeres and an inflammatory response within the muscle (Bakhtiary, Safavi-Farokhi, & Aminian-Far, 2007).

1

Rationale for the Study

DOMS can adversely affect muscular performance, both from voluntary reduction of effort and from inherent loss of capacity of the muscles to produce force (Armstrong, 1984). It is imperative to investigate the effectiveness of possible interventions, to minimize muscular damage and enhance recovery, particularly in athletes. To achieve an appropriate balance between training, competition, and recovery, we must focus our attention on attenuating DOMS. Vibration is one potential intervention to minimize damage and enhance recovery from DOMS (Cheung et al., 2003).

Investigation into the prevention and treatment of DOMS necessitates a preliminary examination into the relationship between DOMS, muscle damage, and inflammation. Recently, Kanda et al. (2013) examined the relationship between DOMS, muscular damage, and inflammatory responses resulting from eccentric exercise in order to observe the mechanisms of recovery from muscle injury. Kanda and colleagues (Kanda, 2013) found that DOMS is inherently linked to the inflammatory response, and in the absence of inflammation, muscular soreness is reduced. Eccentric contractions are known to initiate the inflammatory response (Baird et al., 2012). Therefore, the current study chose to investigate intense eccentric cycling in a population of male recreational runners. The subjects who were chosen all demonstrated a VO₂max of 30 or greater (Gormley et al., 2008). The VO2max value was established to ensure similar cardiovascular fitness in the subject population.

Aminian-Far and colleagues investigated the effects of eccentric exercise on DOMS utilizing whole body vibration (WBV) as a treatment modality (Aminian-Far et al., 2011). WBV elicits an increase in the synchronization of motor unit firing, thereby reducing myofibrillar stress when applied before eccentric exercise (Aminian-Far et al., 2011). Vibration applied before exercise, causes an increase in blood flow, which dampens the effects of exercise through an increase in the aforementioned synchronization. A recent study showed that applying localized vibration before downhill running was an effective therapy for attenuating DOMS (Bakhtiary et al., 2007). Vibration, applied before exercise, elicits an increase in blood flow, thereby dampening the effects of exercise through an increase in the synchronization of motor units. Thus, we hypothesized that applying vibration after eccentric exercise may also have a protective effect on the muscle fibers against further damage. Therefore, our purpose was to address the potential effects of vibration in attenuating DOMS.

Both CK and lactate are known markers of muscle damage that have been found to increase following disruption of the sarcolemma (Cheung et al., 2003). Consequently, DOMS results from this disruption and is associated with the aforementioned biomarkers. Significant decreases in post-exercise CK levels are consistently found after WBV (Imtiyaz, Veqar, & Shareef, 2014). However, WBV can result in many side effects including plantar fasciitis, itchy legs, blurred vision, tinnitus, orthostatic hypertension, and aggravation of soft-tissue and joint injuries (Wysocki, Butler, & Shamliyan, 2011). Therefore, localized vibration may present a unique, and potentially less harmful, approach to explore a method of treatment and prevention of DOMS.

Objective

The purpose of this study was to investigate the effects of localized vibration on muscular damage, following an intense bout of eccentric cycling. Numerous variables were taken into consideration including muscle soreness, perceived pain, creatine kinase (CK), and lactate levels. One of the objectives of this study was to analyze the effects of localized vibration on CK and lactate levels. A second objective was to determine if localized vibration decreases DOMS (measured via pressure algometry) and perception of pain 48 hours post-exercise. A third objective was to determine the effects of eccentric cycling and localized vibration on muscle length and muscle soreness.

My hypotheses were based on the premise that vibration therapy (VT) can be used to attenuate DOMS. VT presents a possible method to address the negative effects of DOMS including muscle-strength loss, soreness, and swelling. My primary hypothesis was that localized vibration therapy via biomechanical muscle stimulation (BMS) would decrease CK levels and lactate levels (24–48 hours) after eccentric cycling. A secondary hypothesis was that localized vibration would decrease perception of pain and enhance recovery (24–48 hours) after a bout of eccentric cycling. A tertiary hypothesis was that a bout of eccentric cycling would result in an increase in muscular soreness and reduction in muscle length, which would recover following localized vibration.

In this document, an analysis of the significance of DOMS is discussed including the etiology, pathophysiology, treatment, and prevention of DOMS. The development of an eccentric cycle ergometer, used to induce DOMS, is outlined. The effect of BMS on muscle damage, following a bout of eccentric cycling, is investigated. Lastly, a look at the effects of eccentric cycling on muscle length and soreness following localized vibration is examined.

CHAPTER II

REVIEW OF LITERATURE

What is Delayed Onset Muscle Soreness (DOMS?)

In 1902, Theodore Hough was the first to reference DOMS and he concluded that this kind of soreness is "fundamentally the result of ruptures within the muscle" (Hough, 1902). Hough stated that when an untrained skeletal muscle performed exercise, it often resulted in discomfort that did not manifest until 8-10 hours post-exercise, and concluded that this "could not be solely attributed to fatigue" (Hough, 1902). Current research strongly suggests that free radicals, which are produced during and after muscular contractile activity, may play a role in DOMS (Close, Ashton, McArdle, & Maclaren, 2005).

Systemically, the production of free radicals results in damage to the skeletal muscle, secondary to the oxidative stress induced by both reactive oxygen species (ROS) and reactive nitrogen species (RNS; Lecarpentier et al., 2014). The correlation between DOMS and muscle damage due to post-exercise free radical production has been demonstrated (Close et al., 2005). Furthermore, free radicals are indicative of cellular injury and death and can lead to a host of chronic illnesses. Free radicals play a physiological role in the function of the sarcoplasmic reticulum by inhibiting the release of calcium at high levels of oxidative stress (Lecarpentier et al., 2014).

The Importance of Treating DOMS

Without proper intervention, the effects of DOMS can lead to debilitating musculoskeletal pain and delayed recovery. DOMS is induced by unfamiliar or excessive exercise that temporally produces metabolites and by-products of tissue damage in the body (Brown, Chevalier, & Hill, 2010). These metabolites result in inefficient blood supply and lack of oxygen in the contracting muscle, leading to pain, muscle weakness, decline of range of motion, and reduction of proprioceptive ability (Cheung et al., 2003). Treatment of DOMS must be timely and effective in order to reduce these associated symptoms.

Etiology of DOMS

Numerous clinical correlates are associated with DOMS including elevations in plasma enzymes, myoglobinuria, abnormal muscle histology, and exertional rhabdomyolysis (Sinert, Kohl, Rainone, & Scalea, 1994). The exact etiology of DOMS is not known, but a number of hypotheses exist to explain this phenomenon. According to Cheung, six hypothesized theories have been proposed for the mechanism of DOMS, including: lactic acid, muscle spasm, connective tissue (CT) damage, muscle damage, inflammation and the enzyme efflux theories; however, the most likely scenario is an integration of two or more of these mechanisms (Cheung et al., 2003).

The lactic acid theory is based on the assumption that lactic acid production continues beyond cessation of exercise (Cheung et al., 2003). The chronic production and accumulation of a noxious stimulus, such as lactic acid, is theorized to result in the subsequent perception of pain even days after exercise (Schwane, Johnson, Vandenakker, & Armstrong, 1983). However, some reports also indicate that lactic acid levels have been shown to return to normal within one hour of exercise, therefore it may contribute to acute pain but not necessarily, the pain experienced in DOMS (Cheung et al., 2003).

The muscle spasm theory of DOMS states that increased resting muscle activation induces a localized, tonic muscle spasm following eccentric exercise (Herbert & Gabriel, 2002). This was thought to lead to a cyclical pattern of localized blood vessel compression, prolonged ischemia, and the accumulation of noxious substances (Herbert & Gabriel, 2002). However, this theory has been tested using electromyography (EMG) and the data have been inconclusive (Abraham, 1977).

The CT damage theory examines the role of CT, which forms a sheath around muscle fibers, in DOMS. This theory states that fast twitch (Type II fibers) may demonstrate increased susceptibility to stretch-induced injury and excessive strain to the CT which may lead to further muscle damage (Stauber, 1989). The content and type of CT differs between muscle fiber types (Stauber, 1989). Fast twitch fibers demonstrate an increased vulnerability to stretch-induced injury, which results in disproportionate strain on the CT (Hough, 1902). Components of mature collagen found in CT include hydroxyproline and hydroxylysine. Post-exercise urinary analysis of these components suggests collagen degradation due to strain injury (Stauber, 1989).

The muscle damage theory of DOMS concentrates on the disturbance of the contractile component of muscle tissue following exercise (Armstrong, 1984). Myofibrillar disruption of the sarcomere is characterized by numerous microscopic lesions in the tissue (Friden & Lieber, 1992). This damage is the result of increased tension, per myofiber, due to a reduction in the total active motor units during eccentric movement (Armstrong, 1984).

Lastly, the inflammation theory, which is based on aspects of the inflammatory response, such as edema, evident following repetitive bouts of eccentric exercise (Francis & Hoobler, 1987). The resulting breakdown of damaged muscle fibers and CT, in addition to the accumulation of bradykinin, histamine, and prostaglandins, attracts monocytes and neutrophils to the injury site (Hasson et al., 1993).

Pathophysiology of DOMS

The etiological theories discussed by Cheung et al (2003), underlies the pathophysiological mechanisms present in DOMS. One such example, the enzyme efflux theory, is based on the assumption that calcium accumulates in muscles following damage to the sarcolemma (Gulick, Kimura, Sitler, Paolone, & Kelly, 1996). The accumulation of calcium is proposed to inhibit cellular respiration, which leads to a decline in ATP regeneration and a resulting degeneration of muscle protein (Armstrong, 1984). Perceived muscle soreness in DOMS stems from the activation of nerve endings surrounding damaged muscle fibers. Eccentric exercise has been shown to produce the greatest amount of damage, including decrements in motor performance at the cellular level (Byrnes & Clarkson, 1986) However, training status of an individual may modulate muscular soreness depending on the activity (Byrnes & Clarkson, 1986).

Exercise intolerance may be the result of a number of different processes (Coudreuse, Dupont, & Nicol, 2004). Differential diagnosis involves confirmation of the source of pain, followed by the potential pathology underlying the myalgia. DOMS generally presents as muscular sensitivity to palpation, contraction, and stretch (Proske & Morgan, 2001).

Some possible explanations exist to describe the etiological mechanisms previously discussed for onset of DOMS including acidosis, site-specific muscle spasms, and microlesions in connective and skeletal muscle tissues (Coudreuse et al., 2004). Evidence further suggests that the progression of DOMS is inherently linked to the inflammatory response, and in the absence of inflammation, muscular soreness is reduced (Kanda et al., 2013). This soreness is a direct result of the regenerative process of muscle repair, which leads to increased muscle mass and hypertrophy (Shoenfeld, 2010).

Eccentric contractions result in greater injury to the muscle tissue, therefore more inflammation and DOMS, than traditional concentric exercise. The role of inflammation in DOMS has not been clearly defined; however, the data suggests that the inflammatory response may be to blame for initiating, amplifying, and resolving skeletal muscle injury (MacIntyre et al., 1995). After a prolonged period of exercise, such as marathon running or after strenuous resistance training, specifically with the involvement of eccentric contractions, numerous functional and structural signs of muscle damage are observed (MacDougall et al., 1998). The etiology of DOMS, which results in elevated lysosomal activity, includes fatigue that is secondary to prolonged exercise, tissue hypoxia, and the formation of free radicals (Appell, Soares, & Duarte, 1992). High intensity eccentric exercise places a large amount of mechanical stress on muscle fibers and can impair muscle function (Byrne, Twist, & Eston, 2004). Training status has been shown to attenuate many clinical signs of fatigue; however, fiber damage occurs nonetheless (Schoenfeld, 2012).

Prevention and Treatment of DOMS

Investigation into the prevention and treatment of DOMS necessitates a preliminary examination into the relationship between DOMS, muscle damage, and inflammation. Recently, Kanda et al. (2013) examined the relationship between DOMS, muscular damage, and inflammatory responses resulting from eccentric exercise in order to observe the mechanisms of recovery from muscle injury. Blood and urine samples were collected pre and post-exercise, with various levels of DOMS reported on subsequent days. Myoglobin concentration significantly increased after exercise as compared with the pre-exercise values. Circulating neutrophil count and migratory activity also increased significantly, whereas there were no significant changes in the other plasma and urinary inflammatory mediators. These results suggest that neutrophils can be mobilized into the circulation and migrate to the muscle tissue several hours after the eccentric exercise and may be involved in the muscle damage and inflammatory processes (Kanda et al., 2013).

Biomarkers and Symptoms in DOMS

In order to examine the effects of different treatment regimens on DOMS, it is important to identify biomarkers of muscle damage. Brown et al. (2010) considered numerous parameters as bio-indicators of DOMS at the hematological level. The results demonstrated various blood chemistry parameters, which were potential biological markers that warranted further investigation (Brown, Chevalier, & Hill, 2010). Analysis and assessment of blood serum and plasma levels is imperative to identify potential biomarkers of inflammation.

The appearance of CK in the blood has been generally considered an indirect marker of muscle damage, particularly for diagnosis of medical conditions such as myocardial infarction, muscular dystrophy, and cerebral diseases (Baird et al., 2012). Serum CK levels increase in the blood following damage to skeletal muscle tissue (Cheung et al., 2003). Eccentric contractions result in both skeletal muscle damage and an increase in CK levels.

CK levels in the blood increase significantly and progressively 24, 48, and 72 hours after bouts of eccentric cycling (Baird et al., 2012). Serum CK levels reflect complex interactions associated with muscle disturbance (Baird et al., 2012). DOMS symptoms can range from muscle tenderness to severe debilitating pain. According to Cheung et al. (2003), alterations in muscle sequencing and recruitment patterns may cause unaccustomed stress to be placed on muscle ligaments and tendons.

Recently, researchers have shown that lactate levels may not be directly linked with DOMS because lactate accumulates in the blood stream immediately following exercise, and clears within 60 minutes, while DOMS does not peak until 24–48 hours post-exercise (Close et al., 2005). However, accumulation of lactate immediately following exercise is an indicator of exercise intensity and thus could be a reliable marker to test the difficulty and performance of exercise.

Recovery From DOMS

Maximizing the recovery time from DOMS is of great importance, particularly in athletes of professional status. A timely recovery will allow an athlete to perform at their highest potential without the limitation of muscular soreness or the inability to produce maximal muscular force. Various modalities are currently being used as integral components of training programs in an effort to obtain a balance between exercise and recovery time. Recovery aimed at enhancing the rate of blood lactate removal has been largely investigated immediately following high intensity exercise in an attempt to reduce the severity and duration of DOMS (Barnett, 2006). The method that is currently being investigated, as a way to expedite blood lactate removal, is through localized vibration.

Biomechanical muscle stimulation (BMS) is a form of localized vibration, which elicits a muscular tonic response. This tonic response stimulates muscle spindles resulting in muscular contractions (Kanda et al., 2013). A recent study by Aminian-Far et al. (2011), investigated the acute effects of WBV applied before eccentric exercise to prevent DOMS in untrained individuals. Volunteers performed six sets of 10 maximal isokinetic eccentric contractions of the dominant-limb knee extensors on a dynamometer. In the WBV group, the stimulus was applied using a vibratory platform (35 Hz) with 100° of knee flexion for 60 seconds before eccentric exercise. The results of this study show that the WBV group exhibited a reduction in DOMS symptoms in the form of less maximal isometric and isokinetic voluntary strength loss, lower plasma CK levels, and less pressure pain threshold and muscle soreness compared with the control group. The data suggests that when administered before eccentric exercise, WBV may lead to a reduction in DOMS and an improvement in muscle recovery. The recovery exhibited through vibration can be explained by the fact that vibration elicits a tonic response and synchronizes motor unit activity, spreading out the resulting damage across a greater surface area, and preventing excessive disruption of sarcomeres (Imtiyaz et al., 2014).

Exercise Modalities in DOMS

A common method of training for maximal strength and flexibility includes exertion with superimposed vibration on target muscles. The existing data from these methods shows that vibration-strength training yields an average increase in isotonic maximal strength of 49.8%, compared with an average gain of 16% with conventional training (Issurin, Liebermann, & Tenenbaum, 1994). The vibration-flexibility training protocol shows an average gain in flexibility in the legs split of 14.5 cm compared with 4.1 cm for the conventional training (Issurin et al., 1994). The application of sinusoidal vibrations has been investigated as a way to activate neuromuscular activity (Aminian-Far et al., 2011). The vibrations elicit activity of muscle spindle afferent fibers, resulting in a tonic reflex. The reflexive mechanism resulting from stimulation of the sensory receptors and Ia muscle fibers, may lead to more efficient muscle fiber recruitment and motor unit synchronization (Bosco et al., 1999).

Vibration in combination with conventional resistance training has been utilized in an attempt to attain greater gains in neuromuscular performance than from conventional resistance training alone. Research in this area suggests that vibration may have a beneficial acute and/or chronic effect on strength and power augmentation. This effect appears dependent upon method of application, amplitude, frequency, and exercise protocols (Luo, McNamara, & Moran, 2005). The vibratory amplitude and frequency determine neuromuscular response, whereby an optimal desired response can be achieved. According to Luo et al. (2005), the method of vibration application (direct or indirect) appears to influence magnitude of amplitude and frequency.

Whole-Body Vibration in DOMS

WBV has been utilized as a therapeutic intervention, which has shown a multitude of positive effects on the muscle tissue. One such effect is the mechanical stretch that is elicited by external stimulation to the muscle similar to that of active maximal stretching. Prolonged muscle vibration increases stretch reflex amplitude, motor unit discharge rate, and force fluctuations (Shinohara et al., 2005). With an acute application of vibration to a relaxed muscle, muscle spindles in humans exhibit a one-to-one response to each cycle of vibration up to ~100 Hz, which can evoke a tonic vibration reflex.

Fagnani et al. (2006) investigated the short-term effects of an 8-week WBV protocol on muscle performance and flexibility in female competitive athletes. The results showed that the WBV group demonstrated significant improvement in bilateral knee extensor strength, counter-movements jumping, and flexibility after 8 weeks of training versus the control group. They were able to conclude that WBV is a suitable training method to improve knee extension maximal strength, counter-movement jumping, and flexibility in a young female athlete.

WBV is an increasingly popular modality of training, especially in sedentary individuals. Significant increases in post-exercise CK levels in the muscle tissue are consistently found after WBV therapy. Delecluse et al. (2003) compared the effect of a 12-week period of WBV training and resistance training on human knee-extensor strength. Isometric and dynamic knee-extensor strength, as well as counter-movement jump height, increased significantly. WBV, and the reflexive muscle contraction it provokes, has the potential to induce strength gain in knee extensors of previously untrained females to the same extent as resistance training at moderate intensity (Delecluse, Roelants, & Verschueren, 2003). The results indicated that significant, yet similar, increases in isometric and dynamic knee-extensor strength were evident in both groups (Delecluse et al., 2003). It can therefore be concluded that WBV, and the reflexive muscle contraction it provokes, can potentially induce strength gains in knee extensors of previously untrained females to the same extent as resistance training.

Vibration has been shown to elicit involuntary muscle stretch reflex contractions leading to increased motor unit recruitment and synchronization of synergist muscles (Bosco et al., 1999). This increase in recruitment of the motor units may lead to greater training adaptations over time (Kosar, Candow, & Putland, 2012). Vibration may also have a protective effect regarding prevention of DOMS. Increased synchronization of motor unit fibers has been shown to reduce myofibril stress during eccentric exercise (Aminian-Far et al., 2011). This reduction in myofibril stress results from the increased synchronization and distribution of impact over a larger number of fibers. Roelants et al. also (2006) reported higher EMG root-mean-square values during WBV compared to a control condition, thus enforcing the motor unit theory (Roelants, Verschueren, Delecluse, Levin, & Stijnen, 2006).

Vibration has also been shown to cause increases in blood flow (Veqar & Imtiyaz., 2014). Increasing circulation will enhance recovery through oxygenation of the affected muscle. However, some disadvantages of WBV include lower back pain, musculoskeletal problems, cardiovascular disorders, neurovestibular disorders and

Raynaud's syndrome (Dandanell & Engstrom, 1986). WBV disadvantages may also include plantar fasciitis, itchy legs, blurred vision, tinnitus, orthostatic hypertension, and aggravation of soft-tissue and joint injuries (Prisby, Lafage-Proust, Malaval, Belli, & Vico, 2008). Determining a proper vibration intervention, while minimizing the possible adverse effects, is of the greatest concern.

Localized Vibration in DOMS

The effects of eccentric exercise on DOMS, after a bout of downhill running, and the associated inflammatory markers therein, have been researched (Schwane et al., 1983). Current literature suggests that vibration therapy (VT) significantly reduces pain from eccentric exercise, decreases histamine levels, increases neutrophils and significantly decreases lymphocytes (Broadbent et al., 2010). It can be deduced from the literature that VT leads to a reduction in muscle soreness and interleukin-6, while stimulating lymphocyte and neutrophil responses, and may be a useful modality in treating muscle inflammation. Research on localized vibration has revealed a significant effect of acute improvements in muscle length (ROM) and perceived stiffness in physically active adults with acute or subacute ankle sprain and hamstring strain injuries (Peer, Barkley, & Knapp, 2009).

Whole-body vibration (WBV) has been found to have an impact on the prevention and treatment of DOMS before exercise (Aminian-Far, Hadian, Olyaei, Talebian, & Bakhtiary, 2011). However, unlike localized vibration, WBV has been shown to have harmful side effects and unknown long-term safety outcomes (Dandanell & Engstrom, 1986). Shinohara et al (2005) compared the influence of prolonged vibration of a hand muscle on the amplitude of the stretch reflex, motor unit discharge rate, and force fluctuations during steady, submaximal contractions. The results indicated that prolonged vibration increased the short-latency component of the stretch reflex, the discharge rate of motor units, and the fluctuations in force during contractions (Shinohara, Moritz, Pascoe, & Enoka, 2005). Thus, a vibration-induced decrease in the force capacity of the muscle was demonstrated.

Lau and Nosaka (2011) tested the hypothesis that VT reduces DOMS and swelling and enhances recovery of muscle function after eccentric exercise. The results showed that, compared with the control group, the treatment group showed significantly less development and faster reduction in DOMS post-exercise. Furthermore, the recovery of muscle length was significantly faster for the treatment group than for the control group. However, no significant effects on the recovery of muscle strength and serum CK activity were noted (Lau & Nosaka, 2011).

Recently, researchers investigating the hypothesis that VT reduces DOMS and swelling and enhances recovery of muscle function after eccentric exercises have produced promising results (Lau & Nosaka, 2011). The study by Lau and Nosaka showed that the vibration treatment was effective for attenuation of DOMS and recovery of range of motion after intense eccentric exercise. This further supports the notion that vibration treatment is an effective method for attenuation of DOMS and recovery of muscle length after eccentric exercise. Building upon the study by Lau and Nosaka, a logical next step is to address localized vibration as a method of DOMS prevention after eccentric cycling.

CHAPTER III

METHODOLOGY

Subjects

A total of 28 recreational runners (18–40 years old) were recruited for this study from the local community of Kent, Ohio. "Recreational runners" were defined as running at least 3 days per week and a VO_2max of 30 ml/kg/min (Pescatello, 2015). A similar study by Bakhtiary and colleagues (Bakhtiary et al., 2007) showed a higher mean CK level in the control group (mean = 195.2 ± standard deviation = 109.2) compared with the vibration therapy (VT) group (116.1±27.8) which was statistically significant (p = 0.001). Utilizing the G*power analysis tool (G*power 3.1.9.2 software), we calculated an estimated total sample size of 28 with a power of .8 and an effect size d of .99.

CK was chosen as the primary variable for the power analysis because the appearance of CK in the blood has been shown as an indirect marker of muscle damage (Baird et al., 2012). Vibration, applied before exercise results in less damage to the muscle tissue, resulting in a decrease in the release of CK in the bloodstream (Imtiyaz et al , 2014). Furthermore, serum CK levels have been found to increase in the blood following damage to skeletal muscle tissue (Cheung et al., 2003). Utilizing these data, we can reasonably assume that our sample size of 28 individuals should be sufficient for the current study.

Prior to enrollment all subjects underwent a comprehensive cardiovascular pre-screening (AHA/ACSM and KSU questionnaire), completed a physician's consent form, and also completed an informed consent form. Individuals with one or more major signs/symptoms of cardiovascular or pulmonary disease, personal history of cardiovascular or related diseases were disqualified from participation in the study as exercising such subjects may pose unnecessary risk. All subjects were evaluated prior to participation in either of these exercise protocols. Before testing, individuals were randomized into one of two groups: control ($n = 14$) or BMS ($n = 14$). The subjects came to the Kent State University Applied Physiology Lab for four sessions within a one-week period. All subjects were instructed to refrain from any physical activity, in excess of their normal routine, in order to control for all parameters assessed.

Localized vibration, via biomechanical muscle stimulation (BMS), was delivered using a device called the Swisswing®. Certain medical conditions precluded the use of the Swisswing®, while other medical conditions required a consultation with a physician or other medical professional. Exclusion criteria included the following: use of a pacemaker, acute inflammation or acute diseases, acute thrombosis (blood clotting), advanced stage osteoporosis, or freshly sutured wounds, joint prostheses and implants of any type, cardiovascular or circulatory diseases, acute hernia, spondylolysis or discopathy, migraine, retinal disease, or epilepsy. If, during the use of the Swisswing® biomechanical stimulation device, the subject felt faint, dizzy, shortness of breath, or discomfort, they were instructed to stop using the Swisswing® immediately, and consult a physician.

Protocol

During the first session, baseline data were gathered including: VO_2 max, a 5-second Wingate power test, muscle length measurement, self-reported muscle pain, pressure algometry and a blood draw to analyze CK level. A 5-second Wingate power test was performed first, which established the target power for the eccentric cycle. Then, a VO_2 max test was performed to establish the subject's maximum oxygen-uptake capacity and determine their ability to perform sustained exercise. Muscle length was measured via range of motion (ROM) at the hip and knee joints of the dominant leg, using a standardized goniometer (de Weijer et al., 2003). DOMS results in a decrease in muscular ROM, therefore a muscle length measurement was taken to determine if the Swisswing® biomechanical stimulation device improved muscle length.

Muscular pain was assessed perceptually using a standard pressure algometer. The algometer was placed at the center of the muscle belly (measured from the tendinous insertion) for the quadriceps, hamstrings and gastrocnemius muscles. The visual analog scale (VAS) was used to determine pain detection and pain threshold (Baker, Kelly, & Eston, 1997). The VAS determined if the Swisswing® biomechanical stimulation device was able to relieve pain, as perceived by the subject, following the eccentric exercise protocol. A Likert pain scale was also used to assess the individual's muscular pain on a scale of 0 to 6, given specific verbal parameters. Lastly, a blood draw was performed to ascertain a baseline CK level.

During the second session, subjects completed a baseline blood-lactate test using a test strip (Lactate Plus Nova Biomedical) before the cycling protocol. Then they performed the 5-minute eccentric cycling protocol on a modified stationary cycling ergometer. After cycling, subjects had a blood sample (5 mL) taken to be analyzed for CK levels and a blood lactate test was also administered immediately post-cycling, using the aforementioned method. Subjects were then instructed to either rest in a chair for 8 minutes (control group), or have 8 minutes of vibration massage on their legs (BMS group). The BMS treatment consisted of four positions for two minutes each at 20 hertz, given on both legs simultaneously: standing gluteals (buttocks resting on drum), standing quadriceps (front of the thigh applied to drum), seated hamstrings (hamstrings draped over drum), and seated gastrocnemius (belly of the calf draped over the drum). During the third session and fourth sessions, subjects returned 24 and 48 hours post-exercise (respectively), to have the following tests repeated: muscle length, lactate, blood draw, algometry assessment, Likert, and self-reported pain assessment (VAS).

Eccentric Cycling Session: Subjects performed a simulated 5-minute eccentric cycling trial on a modified stationary cycling ergometer. The eccentric aspect of this ergometer forced the rider to cycle in a backward motion against the resistance of a motor. The ergometer consisted of a ProForm® recumbent cycle frame, a computerized control mechanism, and a motor developed by Rockwell Automation (Twinsburg, OH).

An increase in speed from 0-40 rpm occurred during the first 15-20 seconds, then subjects were allowed to warm up and become comfortable with the stationary cycle for 2-3 minutes at 40 rpm. After this warm up, the subject was instructed to resist against the 40 rpm for a 5-minute time period. The subject's target power output for the eccentric cycling session was established following a 5-second Wingate power test. The Wingate power test is an anaerobic test that measures peak anaerobic power, as well as anaerobic capacity by pedaling at maximum speed against a constant force.

Control Group: Subjects in the control group were asked to rest in a chair for 8 minutes and quietly read the study protocol (to control for mental imagery).

Biomechanical Stimulation Sessions (as recommended by the manufacturer): The BMS treatment was performed at a frequency of 20Hz and consisted of four bilateral positions for two minutes each. The muscle bellies were targeted in the following groups: standing gluteals – buttocks resting on drum; standing quadriceps – front of the thigh applied to drum; seated hamstrings – hamstrings draped over drum; seated gastrocnemius – belly of the calf draped over the drum.

Assessments: Several methods of assessment were used in this study: VO_2 max, muscle length (unilateral), blood draw, DOMS Visual Analog (VAS) Scale for "muscle pain" (self-reported), pressure algometry assessment (unilateral), and Likert pain scale.

Fitness Assessment Variables

VO_2 max: The protocol consisted of 30 watts at baseline, then increased in increments of 30 watts every minute thereafter until the subjects reached volitional fatigue while maintaining self-selected revolutions per minute (RPM). The VO_2 max protocol was performed on a modified stationary cycle in the Kent State University laboratory. Expired air was collected and analyzed with a Parvomedics metabolic cart (Parvomedics, Provo, Utah) to determine VO_2 max, utilizing the Velotron computer software (Racermate, Chicago, Illinois).

Dependent Variables

Muscle length: Subjects had their muscle length assessed during each session using a standardized goniometer with the subject lying supine on a firm surface (Harvey, 1998).

Muscle length was measured via range of motion (ROM) at the hip and knee joints of the dominant leg (de Weijer et al., 2003). The goniometer was placed at the lateral epicondyle of the knee and the subject was asked to use both hands to support the hip in a 90 degree flexed position. Then, while maintaining the hip flexion, the subject was asked to extend to the limit of motion so that the hamstring was completely stretched (Clarkson, 2005).

For the quadriceps ROM measurement, the subject was asked to sit at the end of the table and grasp the back of their thigh with both hands. They were assisted into a supine position and instructed to pull the thigh toward their chest. The goniometer was then placed at the lateral epicondyle of the knee on the dominant leg (hanging off the table). This position places the quadriceps muscle at full stretch and the hip range of motion was then measured (Clarkson, 2005). Data were collected at baseline, then again at 24 and 48 hours on the dominant leg only. Two trials were performed and the mean value was calculated.

Lactate: Blood lactate levels were tested using a blood-lactate strip and finger prick assessment method during the second, third, and fourth sessions. The hand and finger of choice was determined at the subject's discretion.

Blood Draw: Subjects had their blood drawn at baseline and then following BMS (or resting) on the second session, as well as during third and fourth sessions in the Kent State University Exercise Physiology lab. Blood analysis included plasma CK that was done by Robinson Memorial Hospital hematology lab. Blood draws consisted of a small blood sample (5 mL) taken from the antecubital vein of the arm of the subject's discretion.

Likert Scale: Muscular pain was assessed using a Likert scale, which contained verbal descriptors indicating a level of perceived pain from zero to six. A value of zero indicated "a complete absence of soreness" and a value of six indicated "a severe pain that limits my ability to move". The Likert scale allowed the subject to quantify the amount of pain they were experiencing.

Pressure Algometry and Self-Reported Pain Assessment: Pressure algometry was used to quantitatively assess pain in the quadriceps, hamstrings, and gastrocnemius muscles. The pressure threshold was measured by positioning the pressure algometer, in the center of the muscle belly, at the desired muscle. Anatomical "muscle-belly center" was measured as the halfway point between the origin and the insertion of the muscle in question (Baker et al., 1997). The pressure algometer was then applied, increasing the pressure slowly and continuously (at a rate of 1kg/sec by counting one/one thousand, two/one thousand) and asking the subject to say, "ok" when he/she starts to feel discomfort (Baker et al., 1997). Once the verbal descriptor was stated, the pressure reading on the algometer was recorded. Then they were instructed to acknowledge their level of pain by marking an "X" on the self-reported pain scale once the pressure has reached a pre-determined value of 80N, at which point we ceased applying the pressure (Baker et al., 1997). Muscular pain was measured perceptually using the muscular pain Visual Analog Scale (VAS) for each muscle group (quadriceps, hamstrings, and gastrocnemius). The VAS consisted of a 15 cm standardized line, anchored by two verbal descriptors: "no pain" and "pain as bad as it could possibly be." Subjects were

Table 1

Muscle Classification

	Origin	Insertion
Quadriceps	Anterior inferior iliac spine	Tibial tuberosity
Hamstrings	Ischial tuberosity	Medial/lateral tibial condyle
Gastrocnemius	Medial/lateral femoral condyle	Calcaneus

Table 2

Testing Schedule

Task	Session 1 (T0) Baseline	Session 2 (T1a.) (Pre-Cycling)	Session 2 (T1b.) (Post-Cycling)	Session 3 (T2) 24 hours Follow up	Session 4 (T3) 48 hours Follow up
Blood Draw	X		X	X	X
DOMS VAS scale (self-reported)	X	X		X	X
Algometry Assessment	X	X		X	X
Likert scale	X	X		X	X
Muscle length assessment	X	X		X	X
Wingate/VO$_2$ max test	X				
Lactate test (4 time points)		X	X	X	X
Swisswing® or resting			X		

asked to lie supine on a table and then we asked them to physically draw an "X" where they believe their pain level existed.

Swisswing® Biomechanical Stimulation Device

The instrument used in this study was the Swisswing® Biomechanical stimulation device, a device produced by Swiss Therapeutic Training Products. This device was comprised of a padded drum that oscillated at a predetermined hertz level to provide BMS via vibration to the body tissue. The Swisswing® produced BMS through imitation of physiological tremor.

Statistical Analysis

Data were analyzed using IBM SPSS Statistics 23 software, Chicago, IL. Dependent variables included the following: muscular length, blood lactate, muscular pain, CK level, and muscular soreness (self-reported), with regard to the independent variables of group and time. A 4x2 repeated measures analysis of variance (ANOVA) was used to assess the interaction of time (pre-exercise baseline (T0), post-exercise eccentric cycling session (T1b), 24 hours post-exercise (T2), 48 hours post-exercise (T3) and group (control, BMS) on all the dependent variables. Tukey HSD post-hoc testing was used to evaluate any differences in data. All data were reported as mean±standard deviation. An $\alpha < .05$ is considered statistically significant. Next, we will provide a technical note describing the development of the eccentric cycle ergometer we used to test the above protocol.

CHAPTER IV

DEVELOPMENT OF AN ECCENTRIC CYCLE ERGOMETER

The beneficial effects of eccentric training are well known (Johnson et al., 1976). These benefits include improving muscle function and increasing eccentric strength. A common example of eccentric training, downhill running, involves contracting and actively lengthening the quadriceps muscle (Proske & Morgan, 2001). However, downhill running is not practical for many people who experience pain associated with the high-impact force of this exercise. A practical approach to eccentric exercise, for those who wish to minimize impact on the joints, is eccentric cycling. Eccentric cycling has been shown to be an effective stimulus for improving muscle function (Appell et al., 1992). Thus, the development of an eccentric-cycling ergometer (ECE) is useful to allow individuals to attain the desired results associated with eccentric exercise, without having the deleterious side effects of high impact exercises. This technical note describes the process by which we developed a version of an eccentric cycle ergometer.

The objective of this investigation was to develop, and then use an ergometer, which would maximize efficiency and provide an effective method to perform eccentric exercise. The current study used a similar protocol for the development of the ergometer as Elmer and Martin (2013). The difference was that our ergometer did not use a power meter, but instead used an automated controller developed specifically for governing power output on our ECE. The development of this ECE was necessary in order to test the impact of eccentric training on delayed onset muscle soreness.

28

Methodology

Frame Design

A salvaged ProForm® (Logan, Utah) recumbent cycle frame was used to develop

the ergometer. The recumbent frame (Figure 1) allowed for stable back support while

resisting the motor. The sprocket was bolt-driven with 58 1/8" teeth (Figure 2). A

bracket was welded to the bottom of the frame to hold the motor mechanism, which was

then attached to a transmission system that joined with the ergometer (Figure 3). The

plastic, cushioned seat was held in place by a bolt, and holes were drilled in the frame

approximately one-inch apart to accommodate various user height. The seat was adjusted

by sliding it up or down and replacing the bolt in the desired hole. The seat position was

determined at the discretion of the user, based on what felt comfortable for them. The

subject was instructed to wear tennis shoes, and their feet were placed on the pedals

without any securing mechanism or special footwear.

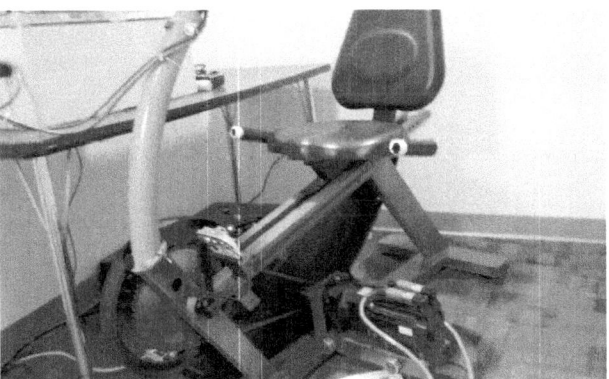

Figure 1. A modified, recumbent eccentric cycle ergometer

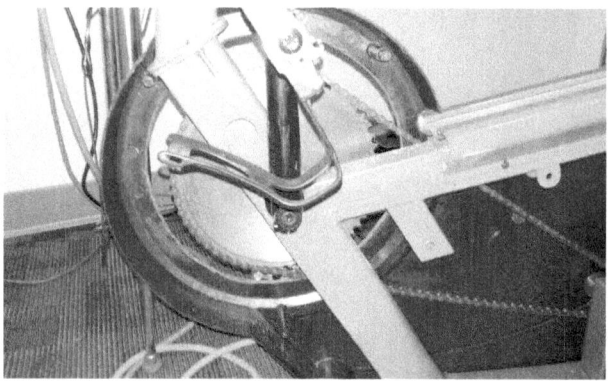

Figure 2. An industrial strength chain connected the gear reducer to the motor unit assembly. The crank spindle was 22mm in diameter, the pedals were platform, and the sprocket was bolt-driven with 58 1/8" teeth.

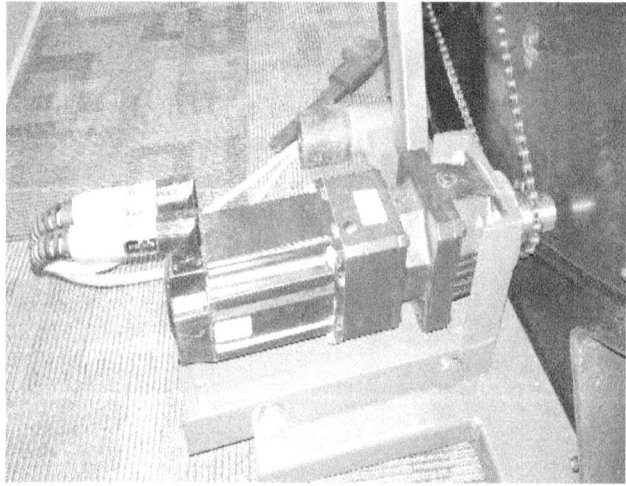

Figure 3. The ServoPro motor unit is attached to the cycle with the assembled mounting bracket.

Motor and Transmission

The essential components of our ECE included the following: recumbent cycle ergometer frame and seat, motor and speed controller to drive the cranks, transmission system that allows for proper pedaling rates and computerized screen that provides feedback to the individual performing the exercise. We used a Servo P series line motor, which allows for torque up to 2000 Nm, developed by Servofit Precision Planetary Gearheads (Maysville, KY). An industrial strength chain connected the gear reducer to the motor unit assembly. The crank spindle was 22mm in diameter, the pedals were platform, and the sprocket was bolt-driven with 58 1/8" teeth.

The motor was controlled using a computerized mechanism developed by Rockwell Automation (Twinsburg, OH). See Figure 4. The computerized control mechanism connected to a monitor that the user could adjust according to speed (RPM) and power output (watts). See Figure 5. The control mechanism governed the movement of the pedals in a backwards direction, producing a force against which the user was instructed to resist. In case of emergency, a stop button was equipped on the side of the panel view computer.

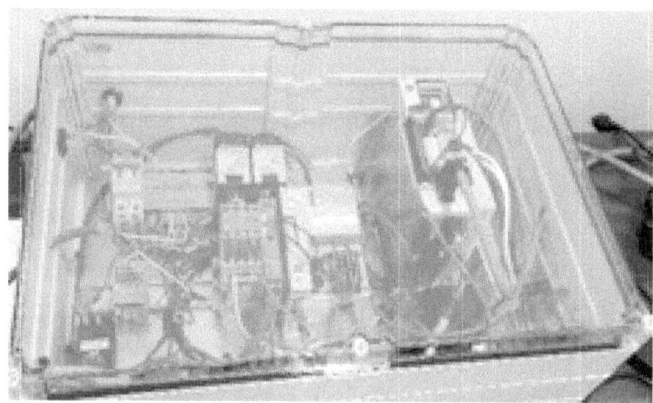

Figure 4. The electronic and electrical components, including the motor drive programmable controller (PLC), network adapter, and power supplies, were mounted inside a hard plastic enclosure. These components were connected to the motor via cables for motor power and control and operator interface.

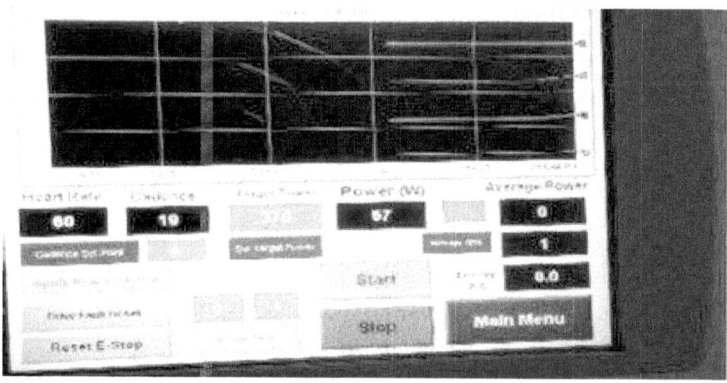

Figure 5. Panel view screen which connects to the computer control mechanism.

Testing Protocol

We had several male subjects (n = 28) test the ergometer by performing a simulated 5-minute eccentric cycling trial. The subjects in this study were 21.39±2.04 years of age, 1.8±.05 m in height, and weighed 77.4±10.5 kg. They had a VO2 max of 39.6±8.7 mL/kg/min and they ran an average of 14.6±15.4 km per week. The eccentric aspect of this ergometer forced the rider to resist the backward motion of the cycle.

Subjects were instructed to mount the bike, and adjust the seat to a comfortable position, they were then allowed to warm up for 2-3 minutes. The eccentric warm up was performed at the testing rate of 40 rpm. The motorized unit was set so that the pedals turned at a 40 rpm rate while subjects were instructed to try and resist the movement, which was sustained for a 5-minute period (McDaniel, Durstine, Hand, & Martin, 2002). A pedaling rate of 40 revolutions per minute, for 5 minutes, has been shown to promote an increase in mechanical efficiency resulting from muscle fibers shortening at their optimal velocity (McDaniel et al., 2002). Subjects were instructed to resist the backward motion as best they could, throughout the duration of the protocol. During this time, each subject's power output was recorded at one-minute intervals (Table 3).

Results

Table 3 shows the power output, during each minute, for the 28 subjects who completed the 5-minute ECE protocol. The subject's goal power output for the eccentric cycling session was established following a 5-second Wingate power test. The results demonstrate each subject's ability to sustain exercise over the 5-minute protocol. "Percent of goal" was determined by taking the average power over the 5-minute

timeframe, and dividing by the goal power. Table 3 shows that 11 out of 28 subjects
(39%) failed to reach their goal power. Of the 28 subjects, 8 (or 28.5%) performed at less
than 95% of their goal.

Table 3

5-Minute ECE Protocol

| Subject # | Power output by time (Watts) | | | | | Goal Power | % of goal |
	1 min.	2 min.	3 min.	4 min.	5 min.		
1	451	477	509	484	501	500.5	96.78%
2	318	343	392	330	518	430.5	88.32%
3	329	378	439	490	522	416	103.75%
4	566	624	538	553	571	396	144.04%
5	305	381	321	380	354	416.5	83.60%
6	398	349	335	292	292	297	112.19%
7	495	525	516	460	458	289	169.83%
8	512	506	395	476	517	496	97.02%
9	524	487	546	342	454	504	93.37%
11	425	453	400	380	530	288	151.94%
12	328	356	382	377	370	389.5	93.09%
13	520	414	433	209	140	330.5	103.84%
14	369	336	392	358	338	504.5	71.08%
15	427	432	406	432	459	273.5	157.66%
16	270	300	342	371	328	294	109.59%
17	412	367	330	319	345	302	117.42%

(table continues)

Table 3 (continued)

5-Minute ECE Protocol

Subject #	Power output by time (Watts)					Goal Power	% of goal
	1 min.	2 min.	3 min.	4 min.	5 min.		
18	222	340	276	242	213	368.5	70.18%
19	415	423	377	355	340	520	73.46%
20	326	367	351	330	323	299	113.51%
21	458	475	476	434	521	371.5	127.27%
22	500	482	427	458	445	467	99.01%
23	599	481	382	401	474	410.5	113.86%
24	321	430	409	457	508	328.5	129.38%
26	424	486	496	488	492	375	127.25%
27	328	356	382	377	370	389.5	93.03%
29	520	414	433	209	140	330.5	103.84%
30	370	305	358	388	357	278	127.91%
31	476	479	481	439	438	392.5	117.86%

Discussion

This technical description outlines the process we used to construct an ECE.

Eccentric cycling can be used in research and clinical settings to cause a phenomenon

known as delayed-onset muscle soreness (DOMS; Baird et al., 2012). The effort to resist

such a force, requires maximal user output, and therefore should greatly damage the

muscles being examined. Construction of the ECE differs from previously constructed

versions (Elmer & Martin, 2013) because ours does not use a power meter to determine power output. Power output was measured with a custom computerized mechanism developed by Rockwell Automation (Twinsburg, OH). See Figure 5. The custom built mechanism avoids the pitfalls that are commonly encountered with power meters including: calibration accuracy, reliability, and validity. The ECE we built focuses on actively lengthening the muscle through eccentric-driven force utilizing a custom-built power measurement device. Eccentric training is more effective than concentric training and therefore should be utilized by individuals seeking increases in muscle hypertrophy (Morgan & Proske, 2004). The ECE trumps other eccentric exercises, such as downhill running, because it allows individuals to avoid the potentially deleterious, high-impact force that running requires. The ECE we developed allows an individual to perform repetitive, high-intensity muscle actions, which may be particularly important in both patient and athletic populations (Baird et al., 2012). In research settings, this ECE protocol can be used to study muscle damage and possible recovery modalities.

In conclusion, we constructed an ECE suitable for research using commonly available parts and some custom fabrication. A limitation of this study was the inability to determine the level of exertion of our subjects. Using a heart rate monitor may have provided a way to better gauge the subject effort. If we equipped the subject with a heart rate monitor, we would be able to calculate what percent of their maximum heart rate they were working at while performing the protocol. Another limitation was the lack of control for the subject's activity level prior to the protocol. If a subject had performed significant physical activity prior to coming in, then they may have been fatigued prior to starting. In addition, stricter requirements controlling for subject fitness level, such as higher VO2 requirements, may have produced better results. This technical note can be useful for researchers who would like to utilize eccentric cycling as a lower extremity exercise modality.

CHAPTER V

THE EFFECTS OF BIOMECHANICAL STIMULATION ON MUSCLE DAMAGE AND DELAYED ONSET MUSCLE SORENESS FOLLOWING A BOUT OF ECCENTRIC CYCLING

Individuals who participate in intense eccentric physical activity often experience delayed-onset muscle soreness (DOMS). DOMS generally peaks 48-72 hours post-exercise and can adversely affect muscular performance from inherent loss of capacity of the muscles to produce force (Armstrong, 1984). Two important biomarkers of muscle tissue damage are the enzymes creatine kinase (CK) and lactate. CK levels in the plasma increase significantly and progressively 24, 48 and 72 hours after bouts of eccentric cycling (Baird et al., 2012). Both CK and lactate levels increase following damage to skeletal muscle tissue, due to disruption of the sarcolemma (Cheung et al., 2003). Researchers have also demonstrated that chronic production and accumulation of lactic acid, results in subsequent perception of pain after exercise (Schwane et al., 1983). The appearance of CK in the blood is considered an indirect marker of muscle damage (Baird et al., 2012). Eccentric exercise is one known method to induce damage to the skeletal muscles, specifically delayed onset muscle soreness (DOMS) (Baird et al., 2012). Recovery from DOMS is of the utmost importance, especially in athletic populations. Attenuating DOMS will allow athletes to perform at a high level without suffering from deleterious effects such as the inability to produce maximal force (Lau & Nosaka, 2011). Lau and Nosaka (2011) found that vibration was effective for attenuation of DOMS and recovery of range of motion after intense eccentric exercise. Vibration resulted in

38

increases in blood flow, which enhanced the rate of recovery. Increasing blood flow leads to expedited delivery of oxygen to the affected tissue.

Veqar and Imtiyaz proposed a mechanism, which may explain the effect of vibration in attenuating DOMS (Veqar & Imtiyaz, 2014). They suggested that a neural adaptation occurs which distributes stress across a larger number of fibers, thus diminishing the effects of DOMS. Vibration has been utilized as a therapeutic intervention that has shown a multitude of positive effects on the muscle tissue. A recent study by Aminian-Far et al. (2011) showed a reduction in DOMS symptoms (when vibration was administered prior to exercise) in the form of less maximal isometric and isokinetic voluntary strength loss, lower CK level, and less pressure pain threshold and muscle soreness compared with the control group. Vibration, when applied to the skeletal muscle and tendon, manipulate the excitatory synaptic input from group Ia afferents onto α-motor neuron (Eklund & Hagbarth, 1966).

Vibration is an increasingly popular modality of recovery that may lead to a reduction in DOMS (Imtiyaz et al., 2014). However, several negative effects have been associated with WBV. WBV has been documented as an occupational hazard linked to lower back pain, musculoskeletal problems, cardiovascular disorders, neurovestibular disorders and Raynaud's syndrome (Dandanell & Engstrom, 1986). WBV disadvantages may also include plantar fasciitis, itchy legs, blurred vision, tinnitus, orthostatic hypertension, and aggravation of soft-tissue and joint injuries (Prisby et al., 2008).

The current study attempted to circumvent these negative effects by utilizing localized vibration instead of WBV. Side effects, such as blurred vision and tinnitus, may be avoidable if an individual limb is treated, instead of the entire body. The current study is also investigating between-training recovery, investigating the effects of biomechanical muscle stimulation (BMS), over three subsequent days.

The purpose of this study was to investigate the effects of BMS on muscle damage following a bout of intense eccentric cycling. The primary hypothesis of this study was that the localized vibration (BMS) group would exhibit a reduction in symptoms of DOMS through a decrease in CK and lactate levels, compared to the control group. One assumption was that lactate and CK would increase following five minutes of eccentric exercise and that vibration would relieve these effects. The secondary hypothesis of this study was that perception of pain would increase following eccentric exercise and decrease following vibration. A tertiary hypothesis was that pain would decrease in the BMS group following vibration, which we measured using a Likert scale (zero – 6).

Methodology

Twenty-eight recreational male runners (control $n = 14$; BMS $n = 14$) completed this study. Both the BMS and control group subjects were similar in age (BMS = 21.6±1.8 years and control = 21.1±2.2 years) and height (BMS = 71.1±1.6m and control = 70.3±2.7m). The BMS group weighed more on average than the control group (BMS = 78.9±10.7 kg. and control = 75.5±9.5 kg.). The BMS group ran more than the control group (BMS = 10.4±14.4 km and control = 7.8±13.7 km). No significant differences were found between the demographic variables of these groups. A study by Bakhtiary and colleagues (2007), showed a higher mean CK level in the non-vibration group

(195.2±109.2) compared with the vibration group (116.1±27.8), when applied before exercise ($p = 0.001$). The sample size for the current study (28 subjects), was estimated based on that study. Utilizing the G*power analysis tool (G*power 3.1.9.2 software), we calculated an estimated total sample size of 28 with a power of .8 and an effect size d of .99. Utilizing these data, we can reasonably assume that our sample size of 28 individuals should be sufficient for the current study.

Subjects: Prior to enrollment, all subjects completed a comprehensive cardiovascular pre-screening questionnaire and an informed consent form. Individuals with one or more major signs/symptoms of cardiovascular or pulmonary disease, personal history of cardiovascular or related diseases was disqualified from participation in the study as exercising such subjects may pose unnecessary risk. Exclusion criteria also included joint prostheses and implants of any type, cardiovascular or circulatory diseases, acute hernia, spondylolysis or discopathy, migraine, retinal disease, or epilepsy. Subjects were counterbalanced into two groups: a control group or a biomechanical stimulation group (BMS).

Protocol: Each subject came to the laboratory 4 times over the course of one week. The following denoted each visit: "T0" (baseline session), "T1a" (pre-eccentric cycling), "T1b" (post-eccentric cycling), "T2" (24 hour follow up), and "T3" (48 hour follow up). Subjects were asked to refrain from any excessive exercise, other than their normal routine, throughout the week. Algometry, muscle length, visual analog pain scale, lactate, CK, and Likert scale were measured during all four sessions. During the first session (T0), baseline data were collected including: VO_2 max, Wingate, baseline

CK level, and various anthropometric measurements such as: height, weight, and age. Before the cycling protocol, a baseline blood lactate test was performed using a blood-lactate strip (Lactate Plus Nova Biomedical) and finger prick assessment (T1a). During the second session (T1), subjects performed a 5-minute eccentric cycling time trial on a modified stationary cycling ergometer. After cycling, a blood sample (5 mL) was taken to be analyzed for creatine kinase (CK) levels (T1). Blood lactate levels were also taken, immediately following cycling (T1b), using the aforementioned assessment method.

After the samples were taken, subjects were instructed to either rest in a chair for 8 minutes (control group) while reading the study protocol (to control for mental imagery), or have 8 minutes of vibration massage on their legs (biomechanical stimulation (BMS) group). The BMS treatment protocol consisted of four positions for two minutes each at 20 hz (on both legs simultaneously): standing gluteals (buttocks resting on drum), standing quadriceps (front of the thigh applied to drum), seated hamstrings (hamstrings draped over drum), and seated gastrocnemius (belly of the calf draped over the drum). During the third (T2) and fourth (T3) sessions, subjects returned 24 and 48 hours post-exercise (respectively), to have the following tests repeated: blood lactate and blood draw (CK).

Fitness Assessment

VO_2 max: The protocol consisted of 30 watts at baseline, then increased increments of 30 watts every minute thereafter until the subjects reached volitional fatigue while maintaining self-selected revolutions per minute (RPM). The VO_2 max protocol was performed on a modified stationary cycle in the Kent State University laboratory. Expired air collected and analyzed with a Parvomedics metabolic cart (Parvomedics, Provo, Utah) to determine VO_2 max utilizing the Velotron computer software (Racermate, Chicago, Illinois). A VO_2max of 30 ml/kg/min was considered acceptable for a recreational athlete (Gormley et al., 2008, 2015).

Workload Assessment Variable

Wingate: The subject's target power output for the eccentric cycling session was established following a 5-second Wingate power test. First, the subject mounted a mechanically resisted bicycle ergometer and was instructed to become familiar by cycling the pedals at a self-selected pace. Once instructed to begin, the subject was told to pedal as fast as they could, against a resistance equal to 10% of their body weight, for a total of 5 seconds. The Wingate power test determined the individual's maximum anaerobic power output, which we used to determine the set resistance level of the ECE. The greater the subject's Wingate power output, the greater the applied resistance of the ECE. The target power output was equal to one-half of the Wingate power output (Elmer et al., 2010)

Outcome Variables

Precision timing was of the utmost importance for collection of the following outcome variables due to diurnal variability. Variability exists because individuals may have a propensity to perform greater amounts of muscle fatiguing actions at certain times of the day over others (Hammouda, Chahed, Chtourou, Ferchichi, & Miled, 2012).

Lactate: Blood lactate was measured using a blood-lactate strip (Lactate Plus lacate meter) and finger prick assessment method during the second (pre and post cycling), third, and fourth sessions.

Likert Scale: Muscular pain was measured using a Likert scale, which contains verbal descriptors indicating a level of perceived pain from zero to six. A value of zero indicates "a complete absence of soreness" and a value of six indicates "a severe pain that limits my ability to move". Measured at the beginning of each session (baseline (T0), pre-cycling (T1), 24 hours post-cycling (T2), 48 hours post-cycling (T3).

Blood Draw: Subjects had blood drawn at baseline (T0), following eccentric cycling (T1) and during third (T2) and fourth (T3) sessions in the Kent State University Exercise Physiology laboratory. Blood analysis included plasma CK which by Robinson Memorial Hospital hematology lab. A small blood sample (5 mL in lithium heparin) was taken from the antecubital vein of the arm of the subject's discretion. Blood was centrifuged at 1500 rpm for 10 minutes.

Testing Protocol

Eccentric Cycling Session: Subjects performed a simulated 5-minute eccentric cycling protocol on a modified stationary cycling ergometer. The eccentric aspect of this ergometer moved the pedals in a backward direction and the rider was instructed to resist the backward motion. The ergometer consisted of a ProForm® recumbent cycle frame and a computerized control mechanism, and motor, developed by Rockwell Automation (Twinsburg, OH). Subjects were allowed to warm up for 2-3 minutes as the cycle increased in speed from 0-40 rpm, then maintained 40 rpm. After this warm up, subjects were instructed to resist the 40 rpm for a sustained 5-minute time period. The subject's target power output for the eccentric cycling session was determined following a 5-second Wingate power test. The Wingate power test determined an individual's maximum anaerobic power output. The target power was determined to be equivalent to 50% of their Wingate power output (Elmer et al., 2010).

Statistical Analysis: Data were analyzed using IBM SPSS Statistics 23 software, Chicago, IL. We assessed the following dependent variables: blood lactate, Likert scale, and CK level, with regard to the independent variables of group and time. A 4x2 repeated measures analysis of variance (ANOVA) was used to assess the interaction of time (T0, T1, T2, T3) and group (control, BMS) on CK and lactate. Demographic variables (age, height, weight, VO2, max power, kilometers per week of running) were compared between the two groups (BMS, control) using independent t-tests. Tukey HSD post-hoc testing was used to evaluate any significance in the data. All data are reported as mean±standard deviation. Statistical significance was set at $P < 0.05$.

Results

We originally recruited 31 subjects, of which 28 subjects completed the protocol (Figure 6). Three of the prospective subjects dropped out before the eccentric cycling phase. Attrition was due to subjects failing to return to the lab after the baseline session for unknown reasons. The BMS group and the control group were randomized equally during the second day of testing (T1).

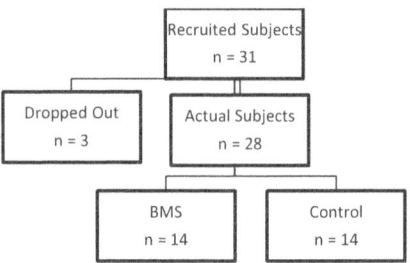

Figure 6. Subjects recruited for the study

No difference was present among the variables (age, height, weight, VO2, km per week, Wingate; Table 4). Subjects in the BMS group were 21±2 years old, 1.80± 0.04 m in height, and weighed 78.9±10.7 kg, average VO_2 max of 38.6±7.4 ml/kg/min, average total kilometers ran per week 10.4±14.4 km, with an average Wingate peak power of 797.7±158.1 watts. Subjects in the control group were 21±2 years old, 1.78± .05 m in height, and weighed 75.5±9.5 kg, average VO_2 max of 40.5±8.7 ml/kg/min, average total kilometers ran per week 7.8±13.7 km, with an average Wingate peak power of 737.9±156.6 watts (Table 4).

Likert Pain Scale

A repeated measures ANOVA revealed that there was no sigificant interaction between group and time ($F(3, 75) = .543, p = 0.362$) for the Likert scale for pain (Figure 7). There was no main effect of group ($p = .655$). There was a main effect of time. ($F(3, 75) = 84.47, p = 0.0001$) and a post-hoc test showed a significant difference ($p = .0001$) for the Likert pain scale. At T2, pain significantly increased compared to T0 and T1, pain remained elevated at T3.

Table 4

Comparison of BMS and Control Group

Demographics	BMS	Control	P – value
Age	21±2	21±2	$p = 1$
Height (inches)	1.80±0.04	1.78± 0.05	$p = .2531$
Weight (kilograms)	78.9±10.7	75.5±9.5	$p = .3821$
VO2max (mL/min/kg)	39.6±7.4	40.5±8.7	$p = .7705$
km/week	10.4±14.4	7.8±13.7	$p = .6286$
Wingate (N)	797.7±158.1	737.9±156.6	$p = .3239$

Lactate

The results demonstrated that there was no significant ($F(3, 75) = .926, p = 0.414$) group-by-time interaction for lactate (See Figure 8). There was no main effect of group ($F(3, 75) = .926, p = .655$). However, there was a significant main effect of time ($F(3, 75) = 3.67, p = 0.025$). Post-hoc tests revealed that there was a significant increase ($p = .016$) between pre-cycling (11a) and post-cycling (11b) for lactate. In addition, there was also a significant decrease ($p = .025$) in lactate immediately after the bout of eccentric exercise (T1b) compared to 48 hours later (T3).

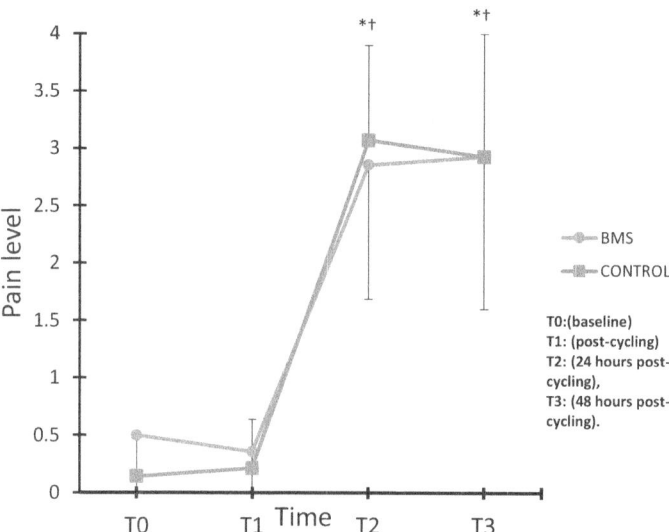

Figure 7. Likert scale for muscle pain across time between groups ($N = 28$). *($p = 0.0001$) significantly different compared to T0. †($p = 0.0001$) significantly different compared to T1.

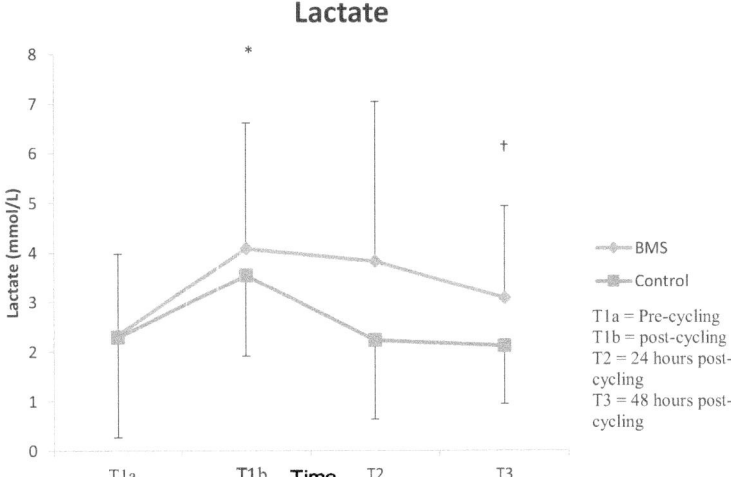

Figure 8. Lactate level across time and group ($N = 28$; $N = 14$ control; $N = 14$ BMS). Lactate increased immediately post-cycling (T1a toT1b) *($p = .016$). Lactate decreased significantly 48 hours post cycling (T1b to T3) †($p = .025$)

Creatine Kinase

The results demonstrated that there was no significant ($F(3, 75) = .175$, $p = 0.284$) group-by-time interaction for creatine kinase (Figure 9). There was also no significant main effect of time ($F(3, 75) = 1.3$, $p = 0.913$) or group ($p = .081$)

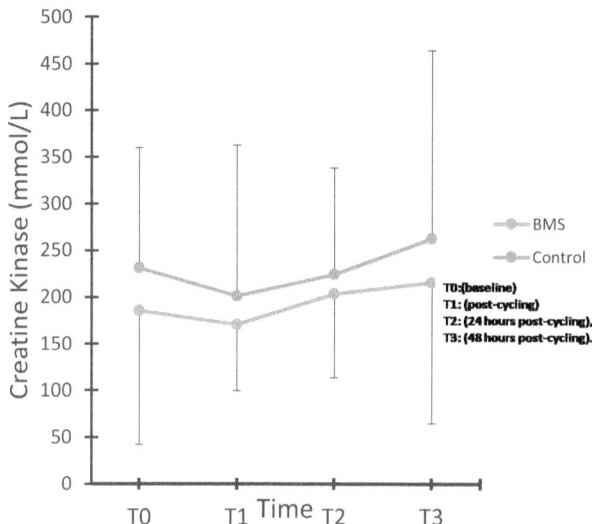

Figure 9. Creatine Kinase level across time. Neither a significant interaction nor a significant main effect of time exists.

Discussion

The purpose of this study was to investigate the effects of BMS on muscle

damage following a bout of eccentric cycling. The hypothesis was that localized

vibration could be used to attenuate symptoms of DOMS by reducing CK, lactate levels,

and pain. Furthermore, the hypothesis that CK levels and perception of pain would

increase following eccentric exercise and decrease following vibration were investigated.

These results are in contrast to a recent study by (Imtiyaz et al., 2014), where muscle pain developed after exercise in all groups but significantly less in the vibration group as compared with control group at 24, 48, and 72 hours of post-exercise. The difference in results is likely because vibration therapy was administered before the eccentric protocol in their study.

Furthermore, the hypothesis that CK levels would increase following eccentric exercise was not accepted because there were no sigificant interactions between group and time for CK. However, the main effect of time suggests that pain increased post-cycling in both groups. These results are in contrast to a recent study by Imtiyaz and colleagues (Imtiyaz et al., 2014), where muscle pain developed after exercise in all groups but significantly less in the vibration group as compared with control group at 24, 48, and 72 hours of post-exercise. The difference in results between the two studies are likely because vibration therapy was administered before the eccentric protocol in their study and it was administered immediately after eccentric cycling in our study.

Blood lactate removal has been investigated following high intensity exercise in order to reduce the severity and duration of DOMS (Barnett, 2006). However, these methods fail to consider circumstances involving between-training recovery, where blood-lactate levels can return to baseline between sessions. Vibration has been utilized as a therapeutic intervention that has shown a multitude of positive effects on the muscle tissue. Vibration has been shown to result in less damage to muscle tissues due to an increase in the synchronization and recruitment of motor unit fibers (Bosco et al., 1999). The subsequent result is a decrease in CK in the blood compared to control group after 48 hours of post exercise (Imtiyaz et al., 2014).

The current study utilized localized vibration and investigated between-training recovery with biomechanical muscle stimulation (BMS) over the course of three subsequent days. The aim of this study was to determine the effects of VT on DOMS and muscle damage. A main effect of time was found between eccentric exercise and lactate level, indicating an increase in lactate immediately post-cycling. Furthermore, a significant main effect of time was found regarding Likert pain scale post-cycling, indicating an increase in quadriceps pain compared to baseline. Lactate, CK, and perception of pain (VAS) were unaffected by biomechanical muscle stimulation.

A limitation of this study was the inability to control for subject effort. The subject was given a pre-determined resistance level, based on their Wingate results. However, the current study failed to control for subject effort. Future research will use this protocol to examine the effects of localized vibration on DOMS, however they will find it beneficial to control for subject effort by equipping the subject with a heart rate monitor.

CHAPTER VI

EFFECTS OF ECCENTRIC CYCLING ON MUSCLE LENGTH AND
SORENESS FOLLOWING LOCALIZED VIBRATION

When a muscle is actively lengthened, sarcomeres are stretched rapidly and uncontrollably (Allen, 2001). Repeated overextension of these sarcomeres results in damage. The muscular injury in delayed onset muscle soreness (DOMS) is the result of eccentric contractions, which cause damage to the muscle cell membrane, thereby initiating a cascade of inflammatory responses (Baird et al., 2012). Muscle soreness is said to begin as early as 6 to 8 hours post-exercise and peaks around 48 hours post-exercise (MacIntyre et al., 1995).

The most common cause of DOMS is eccentric muscular activity (MacIntyre, Reid, & McKenzie, 1995). Eccentric contractions result in greater injury to the muscle tissue, therefore more inflammation and DOMS, than concentric exercise. Vibration has been utilized for years as a therapeutic intervention to decrease muscle soreness by increasing synchronization of motor units and eliciting afferent pathways (Aminian-Far et al., 2011).

The main objective of this investigation was to analyze the effects of localized vibration on muscle length and soreness in the quadriceps and hamstring muscles, following intense eccentric cycling. Muscle fibers with damaged sarcomeres will have a less than optimal length (Allen, 2001). Therefore, it is imperative to determine the effects of eccentric exercise on muscle length and soreness so that we may develop a regimen to deter these deleterious factors. We hypothesized that intense eccentric

53

cycling would lead to an increase in muscle soreness and a decrease in muscle length. Furthermore, we hypothesized that localized vibration would decrease muscle soreness and restore muscle length following intense eccentric cycling.

Methodology

We recruited 28 male recreational runners (control $n = 14$; BMS $n = 14$) for the study. We reached the value of 28 based on a similar study by Bakhtiary and colleagues (Bakhtiary et al., 2007). The Bakhtiary study looked at an important biomarker of muscle tissue damage, creatine kinase (CK). CK levels increase significantly after bouts of eccentric cycling (Baird et al., 2012). In the Bakhtiary study (Bakhtiary et al., 2007), subjects exhibited a higher mean CK level in the non-vibration group (195.2 ± 109.2) compared with the vibration group (116.1 ± 27.8) which was statistically significant ($p = 0.001$).

The sample size for the current study (28 subjects) was estimated based on the (Bakhtiary et al., 2007) study because CK is inherently linked to muscle damage. Utilizing the G*power analysis tool (G*power 3.1.9.2 software), we calculated an estimated total sample size of 28 with a power of .8 and an effect size d of .99. Utilizing this research, we can reasonably assume that our sample size of 28 individuals should be sufficient for the current study.

Protocol

Each subject came to the laboratory four times over the course of one week. The following denoted each visit: "T0" (baseline session), "T1" (eccentric cycling session), "T2" (24 hour follow up), and "T3" (48 hour follow up). The subjects were asked to refrain from any excessive exercise prior to testing. During all four sessions, the following variables were measured: algometry, muscle length, and visual analog pain scale. During the first session, baseline data was collected including: VO_2 max (to establish level of fitness), muscle length, muscle pain (self-reported), pressure algometry, and various anthropometric measurements such as height, weight, and age.

During the second session, subjects performed a 5-minute eccentric cycling time trial on a modified stationary cycling ergometer. Subjects were instructed to either rest in a chair for 8 minutes (control group), or have 8 minutes of vibration massage on their legs (biomechanical stimulation (BMS) group). The instrument used in this study was the Swisswing® Biomechanical stimulation device, a device produced by Swiss Therapeutic Training Products. This device was comprised of a padded drum that oscillated at a predetermined hertz level to provide BMS via vibration to the body tissue. The Swisswing® produced BMS through imitation of physiological tremor.

The BMS treatment protocol consisted of four positions for two minutes each at 20 Hz (on both legs simultaneously): standing gluteals (buttocks resting on drum), standing quadriceps (front of the thigh applied to drum), seated hamstrings (hamstrings draped over drum), and seated gastrocnemius (belly of the calf draped over the drum). During the third and fourth sessions, subjects returned 24 and 48 hours post-exercise (respectively), to have the following tests repeated: algometry, muscle length, and visual analog pain scale.

Subjects

Prior to enrollment, all subjects completed a comprehensive cardiovascular pre-screening questionnaire. Individuals with one or more major signs/symptoms of cardiovascular or pulmonary disease, personal history of cardiovascular or related diseases was disqualified from participation in the study as exercising such subjects may pose unnecessary risk. Exclusion criteria also included joint prostheses and implants of any type, cardiovascular or circulatory diseases, acute hernia, spondylolysis or discopathy, migraine, retinal disease, or epilepsy. Subjects were counter-balanced into two groups: a control group or a biomechanical stimulation group (BMS).

Fitness Assessment Measurement

VO_2 max: This protocol established cardiovascular fitness level for the subjects. The VO2max test consisted of 30 watts at baseline, then increased increments of 30 watts every minute thereafter until the subjects reached volitional fatigue while maintaining a self-selected revolutions per minute (RPM). The VO_2 max protocol was performed on a modified stationary cycle in the Kent State University laboratory. Expired air collected and analyzed with a Parvomedics metabolic cart (Parvomedics, Provo, Utah) to determine VO_2 max utilizing the Velotron computer software (Racermate, Chicago, Illinois).

Power Output Measurement

Wingate: The subject's target power output for the eccentric cycling session was established following a 5-second Wingate power test. First, the subject mounted a mechanically resisted bicycle ergometer and was instructed to become familiar by cycling the pedals at a self-selected pace. Once instructed to begin, the subject was told to pedal as fast as they could, against a resistance equal to 10% of their body weight, for a total of 5 seconds. The Wingate power test determined the individual's maximum anaerobic power output, which we used to determine the set resistance level of the ECE. The greater the subject's Wingate power output, the greater the applied resistance of the ECE. Target

power was equal to one-half of the Wingate power (Elmer et al., 2010).

Outcome Measure Variables

Muscle length: Subjects had their muscle length passively assessed during each

session using a standardized goniometer with the subject lying supine on a firm surface

(Harvey, 1998). Muscle length was measured via range of motion (ROM) at the hip and

knee joints of the dominant leg, using a standardized goniometer (de Weijer et al., 2003).

The goniometer was placed at the lateral epicondyle of the knee and the subject was asked

to use both hands to support the hip in a 90 degree flexed position. Then, while

maintaining the hip flexion, the subject was asked to extend to the limit of motion so that

the hamstring was completely stretched (Figure 10)

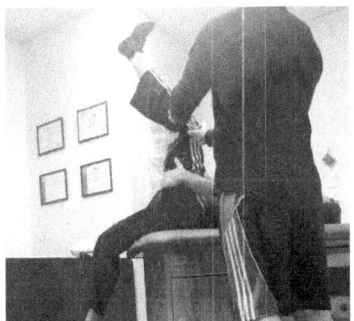

Figure 10. Passive hamstring muscle measurement

The subject was asked to sit at the end of the table and grasp the back of their thigh

with both hands. They were then assisted into a supine position and instructed to pull their

thigh toward their chest. The goniometer was then placed at the lateral epicondyle of the knee on the dominant leg (hanging off the table). This position places the hamstrings muscle at full stretch and the range of motion was then measured (Clarkson, 2005).

The ROM for the hip was measured by having the subject sit at the end of the table and grasp the non-dominant leg while being assisted into the supine position. Then the leg is allowed to relax off the edge of the table while the knee of the non-dominant leg is held in the neutral position (Figure 11).

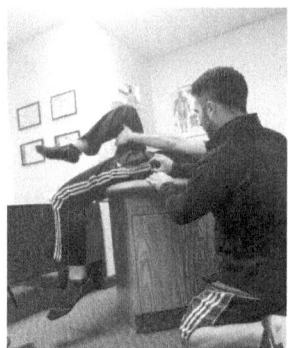

Figure 11. Passive hip ROM measurement

The goniometer is then placed at the midaxillary line along the greater trochanter of the femur and the ROM for the hip is measured (Clarkson, 2005). Data were measured at baseline (T0), immediately post-cycling (T1), then again at 24 (T2) and 48 hours (T3) on the dominant leg only. Two trials were performed and the mean value calculated for analysis.

Self-reported pain scale: Muscular pain was assessed perceptually using a pressure algometer and VAS for each muscle group (quadriceps and hamstrings) (Byrnes

& Clarkson, 1986). The VAS was a 15 cm standardized line, anchored by two verbal descriptors: "no pain" and "pain as bad as it could possibly be." ask the subjects to draw an "X" where they believe their pain level exists.

Pressure Algometry Assessment: The pressure algometer (Wagner FDX, Greenwich, Connecticut) was utilized to quantitatively assess pain in the quadriceps (rectus femoris) and hamstring (semimembranosus) muscles in conjunction with the VAS scale. Pressure detection and threshold were measured by positioning the pressure algometer, in the center of the muscle belly, at the desired muscle. Anatomical "muscle-belly center" was measured as the halfway point between the origin and the insertion of the muscle in question (Baker et al., 1997). The pressure algometer was used by increasing the pressure slowly and continuously (at a rate of 1kg/sec by counting one/one thousand, two/one thousand) asking the subject to say, "Ok" when he/she starts to feel discomfort. The start of "discomfort" varies depending on an individual's perception of pain. Therefore, pain detection varied among the subjects. Subjects were asked to acknowledge their level of pain, by marking an "x" on the VAS scale, once the pressure had reached a pre-determined value of 80N (pain threshold), at which the pressure was ceased (Baker et al., 1997).

Eccentric Cycling Session

Subjects performed a simulated 5-minute eccentric cycling trial on a modified stationary cycling ergometer. The eccentric aspect of this ergometer the rider to cycle in a backward motion. The ergometer consists of a ProForm® recumbent cycle frame and a computerized control mechanism, and motor, developed by Rockwell Automation

(Twinsburg, OH). An increase in speed from 0-40 rpm occurred during the first 15–20 seconds, and then subjects were allowed to warm up and become comfortable with the stationary cycle for 2–3 minutes at 40 rpm. After this warm up, the subject was instructed to resist against the 40 rpm for a 5-minute time. The subject's target power output for the eccentric cycling session was determined following a 5-second Wingate power test. The Wingate power test determines an individual's maximum anaerobic power output.

Statistical Analysis

Data were analyzed using IBM SPSS Statistics 23 software, Chicago, IL. We assessed the following dependent variables: muscular length, muscular pain (pressure algometry), and muscular soreness (self-reported), with regard to the independent variables of group and time. A 4x2 repeated measures analysis of variance (ANOVA) was used to assess the interaction of time (T0, T1, T2, and T3) and group (control, BMS) on the variables of muscle length, pressure algometry, and muscular pain.

Results

Of the 31 recruited subjects, 28 subjects completed this research ($n = 28$, Figure 12). Three subjects dropped out of the study before the second session (T1) and did not return to the lab for undisclosed reasons. The BMS group and the control group were randomized equally.

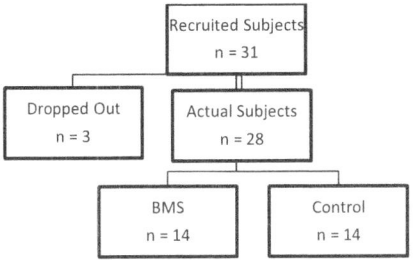

Figure 12. Subjects recruited for the study

Subjects in the BMS group were 21±2 years old, 1.80± 0.04 m in height, and weighed 78.9±10.7 kg, average VO_2 max of 38.6±7.4 ml/kg/min, average total kilometers ran per week 10.4±14.4 km, with an average Wingate peak power of 797.7±158.1 watts. Subjects in the control group were 21±2 years old, 1.78± .05 m in height, and weighed 75.5±9.5 kg, average VO_2 max of 40.5±8.7 ml/kg/min, average total kilometers ran per week 7.8±13.7 km, with an average Wingate peak power of 737.9±156.6 watts.

Algometry

Hamstring: There was no significant interaction ($F(3, 78) = 1.419$, $p = 0.244$) between group and time for pain detection in the hamstring (Figure 13). There was also no main effect of time ($F(3, 78) = .700$, $p = 0.555$) or group ($p = 0.363$)

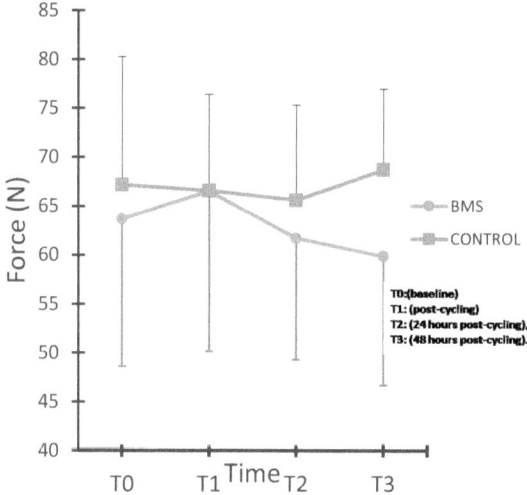

Algometry Hamstring

Figure 13. Pressure algometry pain detection (N) at the hamstring muscle across time. Neither a significant interaction nor a significant main effect of time (or group) exists.

Quadriceps: There was no significant interaction ($F(3, 78) = .853$, $p = 0.853$) for pain detection in the quadriceps (Figure 14). There was also no main effect of time ($F(3, 78) = 1.659$, $p = 0.183$) or group ($p = .785$)

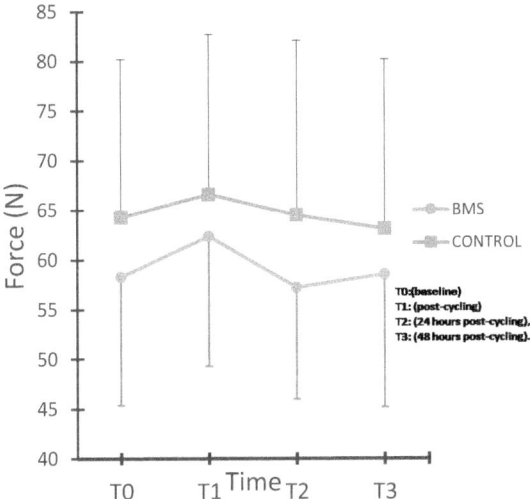

Figure 14. Pressure algometry pain detection (N) in the quadriceps muscle across time. Neither a significant interaction nor a significant main effect of time (or group) exists.

Muscle Length

Quadriceps: There was no significant interaction between group and time ($F(3, 78) = .209$, $p = 0.853$) for muscle length in the quadriceps (Figure 15). There was also no main effect of time ($F(3, 78) = 1.76$, $p = 0.160$) or group ($p = .628$)

64

Muscle Length Quadriceps

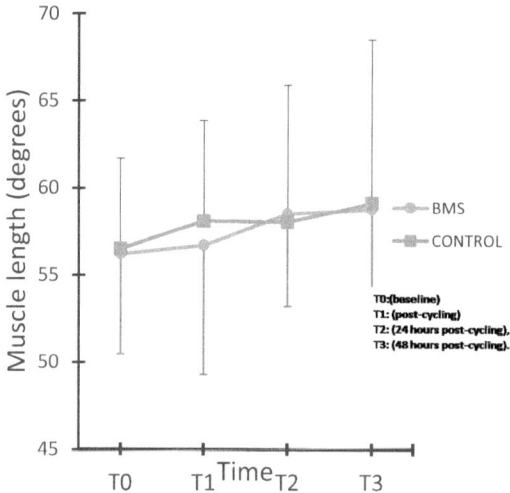

Figure 15. Muscle length measurement (in degrees) of the quadriceps muscle. Neither a significant interaction nor a significant main effect of time (or group) exists.

Hamstring: There was no significant interaction ($F(3, 78) = .778, p = 0.510$)

between group and time for muscle length in the hamstrings (Figure 16). There was also

no main effect of time ($F(3, 78) = 1.16, p = 0.330$) or group ($p = .210$)

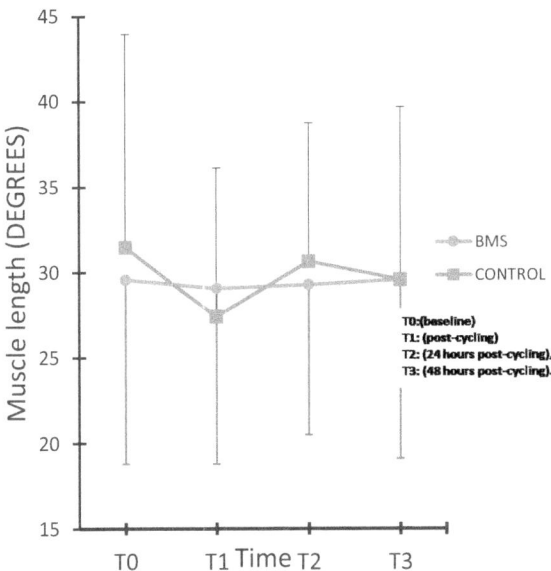

Muscle length Hamstring

Figure 16. Muscle length measurement (degrees) of the hamstring muscle. Neither a significant interaction nor a significant main effect of time (or group) exists.

Visual Analog Scale

Pain Detection Hamstring: There was no significant interaction ($F(3, 78) = 1.08$, $p = 0.363$) between group and time for pain detection in the hamstrings (Figure 17). There was also no main effect of time ($F(3, 78) = .958$, $p = 0.417$) or group ($p = .337$)

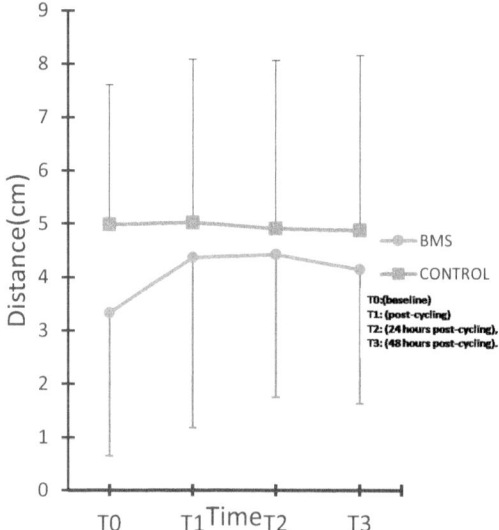

Figure 17. Visual analog scale pain detection of the hamstring muscle. Neither a significant interaction nor a significant main effect of time (or group) exists.

Pain Threshold Hamstring: There was no significant interaction ($F(3, 78) = .880$, $p = 0.39$) for pain threshold in the hamstrings (Figure 18). There was also no main effect of time ($F(3, 78) = .912$, $p = 0.439$) or group ($p = .455$)

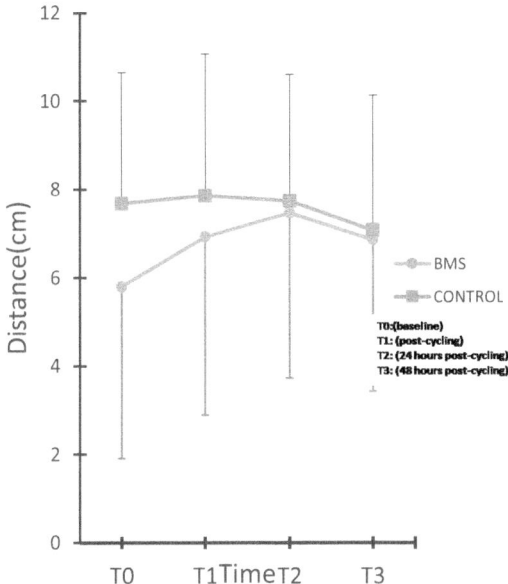

Figure 18. Visual analog scale pain threshold of the hamstring muscle (cm). Neither a significant interaction nor a significant main effect of time (or group) exists.

Pain Detection Quadriceps: There was no significant interaction ($F(3, 78) = 1.223$ $p = 0.307$) between group and time for pain detection in the quadriceps (Figure 19). There was also no main effect of time ($F(3, 78) = 1.28, p = 0.287$) or group ($p = .316$)

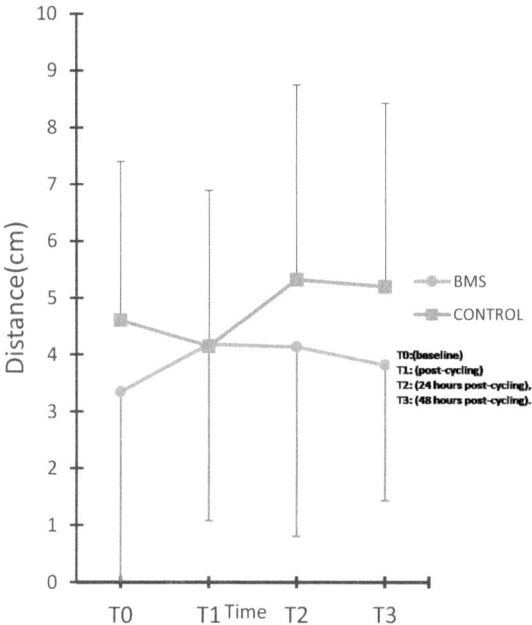

Figure 19. Visual analog scale pain detection of the quadriceps muscle (cm). Neither a significant interaction nor a significant main effect of time (or group) exists.

Pain Threshold Quadriceps: There was no significant ($F(3, 78) = 1.092, p = 0.489$) group-by-time interaction for pain threshold in the quadriceps (Figure 18). Post-hoc tests determined a significant ($F(3, 78) = 3.02, p = 0.043$) main effect of time which shows that both groups experienced an increase in pain 24 hours post-cycling (T2) versus pre-cycling (T1). There was no main effect of group ($p = .816$)

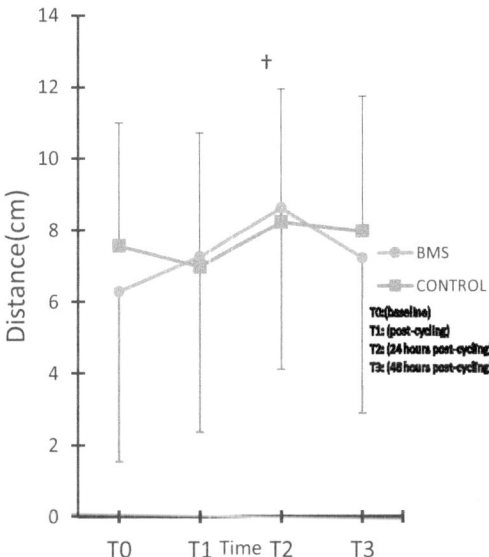

Figure 20. Visual analog scale pain threshold of the quadriceps muscle (cm). Main effect of time (†$p = .043$) both groups experienced an increase in pain 24 hours post-cycling (T2) versus pre-cycling (T1)

Discussion

Vibration has been shown to increase muscle spindle activity and enhance motor unit synchronization, which may optimize neuromuscular facilitation (Imtiyaz et al., 2014). Our investigation sought to analyze the effects of localized vibration on muscle length and soreness in the quadriceps and hamstring muscles, following intense eccentric cycling. We can conclude that both the control group, and the BMS group, experienced an increase in pain in the quadriceps muscle after a bout of intense eccentric cycling. These data confirm previous data by Elmer et al., 2010, that demonstrated similar results utilizing eccentric cycling to induce quadriceps pain. It is commonly known that intense eccentric exercise induces not only changes in muscle length, but also changes in muscle damage (Morgan & Proske, 2004). Furthermore, the extent of such damage can be dependent on the muscle length (Aminian-Far, et al., 2011). The extent to which eccentric exercise and subsequent muscle soreness affects a task may vary depending on the rate of force development of that task (Crameri et al., 2007).

Eccentric exercise and subsequent soreness are known to affect motor output and muscle length. This study examined the effect of eccentric exercise on soreness and length of the muscle, following localized vibration. The results indicate that muscular pain threshold is increased in the quadriceps following intense eccentric cycling on a modified stationary ergometer. A limitation of this study was that we were unable to control for subject effort on the eccentric cycle ergometer. The subject was given a pre-determined resistance level, based on their Wingate results. However, the amount of effort by which the subject resisted the ergometer was not controlled for. This could have been resolved if we had equipped the subject with a heart rate monitor. Another limitation was that we were unable to control for subject activity outside the lab. Future research will use this protocol to examine the effects of eccentric cycling on muscle soreness, but they may find it beneficial use electromyography to determine the exact muscle group being affected and can focus treatment specifically on that individual quadriceps muscle.

CHAPTER VII

SUMMARY

Delayed onset muscle soreness (DOMS) is musculoskeletal pain resulting from intense physical activity. Eccentric cycling is one commonly used modality by which DOMS can be elicited. To our knowledge, few studies have investigated the effects of localized vibration on biomarkers and symptoms of DOMS following intense eccentric cycling. The purpose of this investigation was threefold: to analyze the effects of localized vibration on creatine kinase (CK) and lactate levels following intense eccentric cycling, to determine if localized vibration decreases DOMS and perception of pain 48 hours post-exercise, and to determine the effects of eccentric cycling on muscular length and muscular soreness following localized vibration.

The results of this study proved significance with regard to a main effect of time in three different variables. Pain threshold, measured via pressure algometry, increased in the quadriceps muscles for both groups immediately following a bout of eccentric cycling. Lactate level increased immediately post-cycling, versus pre-cycling, in both groups. Lactate level also decreased in both groups 48 hours post-cycling. Finally, Likert pain scores increased in both groups, post cycling versus pre-cycling. These results indicate that pain threshold, perceived pain, and lactate all increased because of the eccentric cycling protocol. None of the variables we investigated were affected by the vibration treatment.

Localized vibration therapy, via biomechanical muscle stimulation (BMS), had no impact on CK, lactate, or perception of pain after a bout of eccentric cycling,

Furthermore, the eccentric cycling protocol did not significantly increase muscular pain detection, nor did it result in a decrease in muscle length. These variables may have been unaffected due several reasons. Subject vibration treatment occurred post-cycling, rather than pre-cycling, which may have accounted for the results we achieved. Vibration, when applied before exercise, has been shown to have a protective effect on the muscle tissue by increasing blood flow, as well as stimulating recruitment of nearby motor units (Bosco et al., 1999). Several research studies have utilized vibration before an eccentric cycling protocol, with much success. A previous study showed that applying localized vibration before exercise was an effective therapy for attenuating DOMS (Bakhtiary et al., 2007). Vibration, applied before exercise, elicits an increase in blood flow, thereby dampening the effects of exercise through an increase in the synchronization of motor units

Another reason for our lack of significant results could be due to the inability to control for subject effort. A possible solution could be to equip the subject with a heart rate monitor to ensure that they are cycling at a high intensity. Furthermore, our results may have been skewed because we did not control for the activity level of the subject before or after the protocol. If the subject engaged in physical activity, especially involving their lower extremities, our results could have been significantly altered. Controlling for fitness level was one aspect of our recruitment protocol. However, we did not specify the extent of physical fitness; rather we simply required that the subject met a level considered to "recreational". The difference in fitness level may have explained the large variance in Wingate power output ability. Lastly, our data collection did not occur until approximately 20 minutes post-exercise, which may have allowed CK and lactate levels to recover, thus skewing our results.

Future research will use this protocol to examine the effects of eccentric cycling on muscle soreness. However, they will find it beneficial to modify several aspects of the protocol including: using more specific fitness requirements during recruitment, equipping subject's with a heart rate monitor, using electromyography to determine the specific quadriceps muscle group affected, and collecting data immediately post-exercise.

APPENDICES

APPENDIX A

ILIOPSOAS DATA

Appendix A

Iliopsoas Data

Muscle length

Iliopsoas: There was no significant interaction ($F(3, 78) = .655$, $p = 0.582$) for muscle length in the iliopsoas muscle (Figure 21). There was also no main effect of time ($F(3, 78) = 1.9$, $p = 0.135$) or group ($p = .182$)

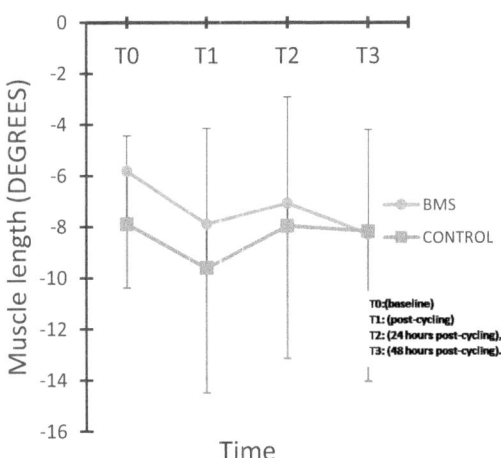

Muscle length measurement (degrees) of the iliopsoas muscle.

APPENDIX B

GASTROCNEMIUS DATA

Visual Analog Scale

Gastrocnemius Pain Detection: There was no significant interaction ($F(3, 78)$ = .328, p = 0.322) for pain detection in the gastrocnemius muscle (Figure 20). There was also no main effect of time ($F(3, 78)$ = 2.78, p = 0.065) or group (p = .257)

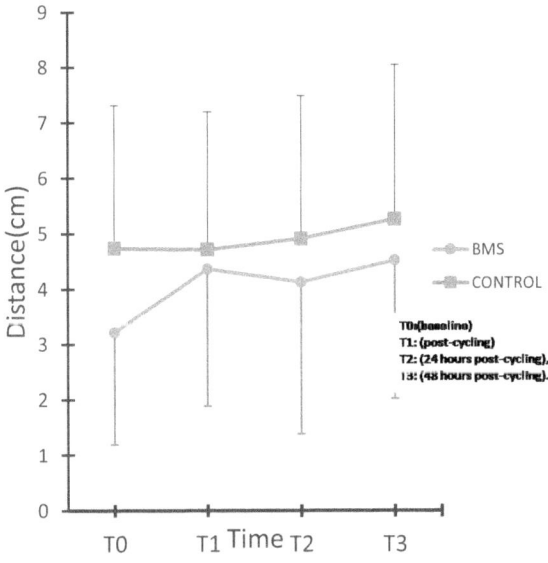

Visual analog scale pain detection of the gastrocnemius muscle (cm). A main effect of time (p = .034) demonstrates an increase in pain threshold for both groups post-cycling.

Gastrocnemius Pain Threshold: There was no significant interaction ($F(3, 78) =$ .096, $p = 0.962$) for pain threshold in the gastrocnemius muscle (Figure 21). There was however a main effect of time ($F(3, 78) = 3.04$, $p = 0.034$). There was no main effect of group ($p = .887$)

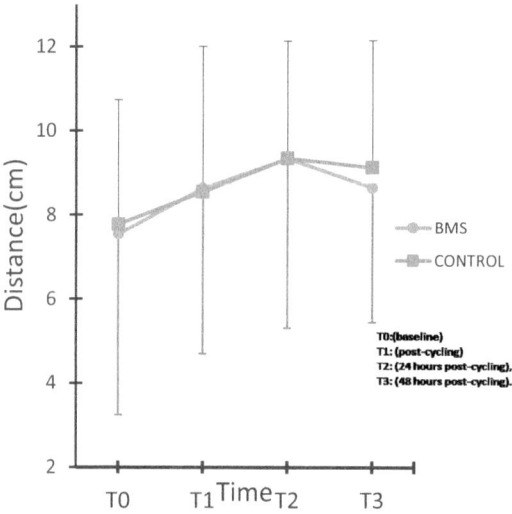

Visual analog scale pain threshold of the gastrocnemius muscle (cm).

Pressure Algometry

Gastrocnemius: There was no significant interaction ($F(3, 78) = .678, p = 0.061$)

for pain detection in the gastrocnemius (Figure 24). There was also no main effect of

time ($F(3, 78) = 2.557, p = 0.568$) or group ($p = .418$).

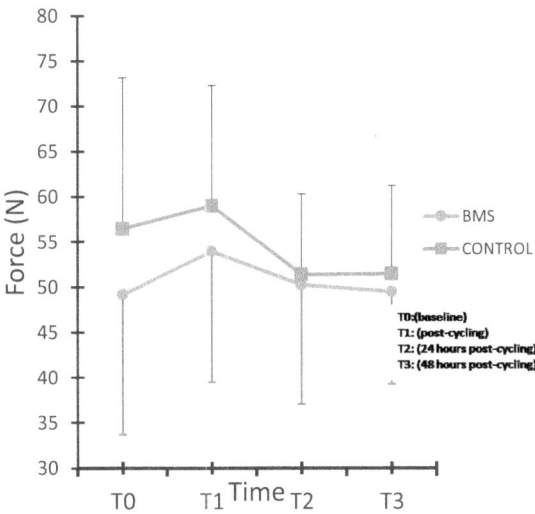

Pressure algometry pain detection (N) in the gastrocnemius muscle across time.

APPENDIX C

LETTER OF CONSENT

Appendix C

Letter of Consent

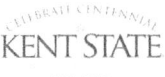

KENT STATE

Informed Consent to Participate in a Research Study

Study Title: ANALYZING THE EFFECTS OF LOCALIZED VIBRATION ON DELAYED ONSET MUSCLE SORENESS FOLLOWING INTENSE ECCENTRIC CYCLING
Principal Investigators: Fredrick Peters, John McDaniel, PhD and Angela L. Ridgel, PhD

You are being invited to participate in a research study. This consent form will provide you with information on the research project, what you will need to do, and the associated risks and benefits of the research. Your participation is voluntary. Please read this form carefully. It is important that you ask questions and fully understand the research in order to make an informed decision. You will receive a copy of this document to take with you.

Purpose
The purpose of this study is to examine the effect of the Swisswing® (BMS) unit – a localized vibration machine – on delayed onset muscle soreness (DOMS) following a bout of intense cycling exercise.

Procedures
If you chose to participate then you was asked to visit the lab for four sessions over a one week period. You will then be randomly placed into one of two groups: 1) control (no therapy) or 2) biomechanical muscle stimulation (BMS). At the first session, your muscle length, cardiovascular fitness, muscle pain and soreness was examined. In addition, a small blood sample (5 milliliters, about 1 teaspoon) was taken from your arm. During the second session, you will complete a 5-minute intense cycling session. If you are in the control group, you was asked to rest in a chair for about 10 minutes. If you are assigned to the BMS group, you will have a 10 minutes vibration massage on your legs. After this 10 minute time period, another small blood draw and a muscle pain assessment was completed you was asked come in 24 and 48 hours after exercise to have these tests repeated (blood draw and pain assessments).

Benefits
Localized vibration may temporarily decrease muscle stiffness and pain and may increase muscle length in the legs after intense cycling exercise. This study will also provide general information about the effectiveness of the Swisswing® Biomechanical stimulation device following muscle damage.

Risks and Discomforts
There are minor risks or discomforts associated with this study such as muscles soreness or pain, bruising from the blood draw and skin tingling. Every effort was made to minimize risks. If you

83

experience any sensation that is unusual or uncomfortable, please tell the staff and they will stop the session.
Medical treatment by the University Health Center is provided only to currently registered students. Please be advised that for all other injuries, emergency services was called for those occurring on the Kent State University campus. You or your medical insurance was billed for this service. No other medical treatment or financial compensation for injury from participation in this research project is available.

Privacy and Confidentiality
Your study related information was kept confidential within the limits of the law. Any identifying information was kept in a secure location and only the researchers will have access to the data. Research subjects will not be identified in any publication or presentation of research results; only aggregate data was used. Your research information may, in certain circumstances, be disclosed to the Institutional Review Board (IRB), which oversees research at Kent State University, or to certain federal agencies. Confidentiality may not be maintained if you indicate that you may do harm to yourself or others.

Compensation
You will receive a gift card for $10 per session ($40 total if study is complete).

Voluntary Participation
Taking part in this research study is entirely up to you. You may choose not to participate or you may discontinue your participation at any time without penalty or loss of benefits to which you are otherwise entitled. You was informed of any new, relevant information that may affect your health, welfare, or willingness to continue your study participation.

Contact Information
If you have any questions or concerns about this research, you may contact Angela L. Ridgel, PhD at 330.672-7495. This project has been approved by the Kent State University Institutional Review Board. If you have any questions about your rights as a research subject or complaints about the research, you may call the IRB at 330.672.2704.

Consent Statement and Signature
I have read this consent form and have had the opportunity to have my questions answered to my satisfaction. I voluntarily agree to participate in this study. I understand that a copy of this consent was provided to me for future reference.

_____   _____
Subject Signature   **Date**

APPENDIX D

AUTHORIZATION TO USE OR DISCLOSE INFORMATION

Authorization to Use or Disclose Information

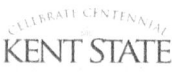

KENT STATE

Authorization to Use or Disclose Health Information that Identifies You for a Research Study

Study Title: ANALYZING THE EFFECTS OF LOCALIZED VIBRATION ON DELAYED ONSET MUSCLE SORENESS FOLLOWING INTENSE ECCENTRIC CYCLING

Principal Investigators: Fredrick Peters, Angela L. Ridgel, PhD

If you sign this document, you give permission to the Department of Exercise
Physiology at Kent State University to use or disclose your health information that identifies you for the aforementioned research study.
The health information that we may use or disclose for this research includes medical records, results of physical examinations, medical history, lab tests, and certain health information indicating or relating to a particular condition. This includes the health history questionnaire that you completed previously upon joining the research project.

The health information listed above may be used by and/or disclosed to the
Department of Exercise Physiology at Kent State University:
Dr. Angela Ridgel, Exercise Physiology
Fredrick Peters, Exercise Physiology

The Department of Exercise Physiology at Kent State University is required by law to protect your health information. By signing this document, you authorize the Department of Exercise Physiology at Kent State University to use and/or disclose your health information for this research. Those persons who receive your health information may not be required by Federal privacy laws (such as the Privacy Rule) to protect it and may share your information with others without your permission, if permitted by laws governing them.
Please note that you may change your mind and revoke this authorization at any time, except to the extent that the Department of Exercise Physiology at Kent
State University has already acted based on this Authorization. To revoke this authorization, you must write to: ATTN: Dr. Angela Ridgel, Exercise Science
Laboratory, 163F MACC Annex, Kent State University, Kent OH 44224.
This authorization does not have an expiration date.

Print Name _____

_____
Signature Date

APPENDIX E

HEALTH HISTORY FORM

Appendix E

Health History Form

KENT STATE UNIVERSITY
APPLIED PHYSIOLOGY RESEARCH LAB
HEALTH HISTORY

Thank you for volunteering to be a subject for a study to be conducted in the Applied Physiology Research Laboratory. Some of the tests used in our experiments require that you perform strenuous exercise. Consequently, it is important that we have an accurate assessment of your past and present health status to assure that you have no medical conditions that would make the tests especially dangerous for you. Please complete the health history as accurately as you can.

THIS MEDICAL HISTORY IS CONFIDENTIAL AND WAS SEEN ONLY BE THE INVESTIGATORS AND KENT STATE UNIVERSITY HEALTH CENTER PERSONNEL

Name_____

Date____/____/____

Date of Birth____/____/____   Present Age_____yrs

Ethnic Group: ____ White
             ____ African American
             ____ Hispanic
             ____ Asian
             ____ Pacific Islands
             ____ American Indian
             ____ Other_____

HOSPITALIZATIONS AND SURGERIES
If you have ever been hospitalized for an illness or operation, please complete the chart below. Do not include normal pregnancies, childhood tonsillectomy, or broken bones.

YEAR_____

OPERATIONS OR ILLNESS

_____

YEAR_____

OPERATIONS OR ILLNESS

YEAR_____

OPERATIONS OR ILLNESS

Are you under long-term treatment for a protracted disease, even if presently not taking medication? [ ] Yes [ ] No
If Yes, explain:_____

MEDICATIONS
Please list all medications that you have taken within the past 8 weeks: (Include prescriptions, vitamins, over-the-counter drugs, nasal sprays, aspirins, birth control pills, etc.)
Check this box [ ] if you have not taken any medication.

MEDICATION_____
    DOSE_____
REASON FOR TAKING THIS

MEDICATION_____
    DOSE_____
REASON FOR TAKING THIS

MEDICATION_____
    DOSE_____
REASON FOR TAKING THIS

MEDICATION_____
    DOSE_____
REASON FOR TAKING THIS

_____

_____

ALLERGIES
Please list all allergies you have (include pollen, drugs, alcohol, food, animals, etc.)
Check this box [ ] if you have no allergies.
1._____
2._____
3._____
4._____

When was the last time you were "sick"? (e.g. common cold, flu, fever, etc.)

_____

PROBLEMS AND SYMPTOMS
Place an X in the box next to any of the following problems or symptoms that you have had:

General
[ ] Mononucleosis
      If yes, when_____
[ ] Excessive fatigue
[ ] Recent weight loss while not on a diet
[ ] Recent weight gain
[ ] Thyroid disease
[ ] Fever, chills, night sweats
[ ] Diabetes
[ ] Arthritis
[ ] Sickle Cell Anemia
[ ] Heat exhaustion or heat stroke
[ ] Recent sunburn

Heart and Lungs
[ ] Abnormal chest x-ray
[ ] Pain in chest (persistent and/or exercise related)
[ ] Heart attack
[ ] Coronary artery disease
[ ] High blood pressure
[ ] Rheumatic fever
[ ] Peripheral vascular disease
[ ] Blood clots, inflammation of veins (phlebitis)

[ ] Asthma, emphysema, bronchitis
[ ] Shortness of breath
    [ ] At rest
    [ ] On mild exertion
[ ] Discomfort in chest on exertion
[ ] Palpitation of the heart; skipped or extra beats
[ ] Heart murmur, click
[ ] Other heart trouble
[ ] Lightheadedness or fainting
[ ] Pain in legs when walking
[ ] Swelling of the ankles
[ ] Need to sleep in an elevated position with several pillows

G-U SYSTEM
[ ] Get up at night to urinate frequently
[ ] Frequent thirst
[ ] History of kidney stones, kidney disease

G.I. TRACT
[ ] Eating disorder (e.g. anorexia, bulimia)
[ ] Yellow jaundice
    If yes, when_____
[ ] Hepatitis
    If yes, when_____
[ ] Poor appetite
[ ] Frequent indigestion or heartburn
[ ] Tarry (black) stool
[ ] Frequent nausea or vomiting
[ ] Intolerance of fatty foods
[ ] Changes in bowel habits
[ ] Persistent constipation
[ ] Frequent diarrhea
[ ] Rectal bleeding
[ ] Unusually foul smelling or floating stools
[ ] Pancreatitis

Nervous System
[ ] Alcohol problem
[ ] Alcohol use
    If yes, how many drinks ingested per week _____
[ ] Frequent or severe headaches
[ ] Stroke
[ ] Attacks of staggering, loss of balance, dizziness
[ ] Persistent or recurrent numbness or tingling of hands or feet

[ ] Episode of difficulty in talking
[ ] Prolonged periods of feeling depressed or "blue"
[ ] Difficulty in concentrating
[ ] Suicidal thoughts
[ ] Have had psychiatric help

Have you ever passed out during or after exertion?   YES   NO

Do you have a family history of coronary artery disease   YES   NO
        If yes, Who? (Grandparents, parents, siblings, uncles, and aunts)

Are there any other reasons not mentioned above that you feel you should not
participate in this research study?   YES   NO

Do you currently smoke cigarettes?   YES   NO

Do you currently use any smokeless tobacco products?   YES   NO

APPENDIX F

PRE-EXERCISE MEDICAL EVALUATION

Pre-Exercise Medical Evaluation

PRE-EXERCISE MEDICAL EVALUATION
AHA/ACSM Health/Fitness Facility Pre-participation Screening Questionnaire

Assess your health status by checking all true statements:

Have you had:

History:
_____ A heart attack.
_____ Heart surgery.
_____ Cardiac catheterization.
_____ Angioplasty or stent.
_____ Pacemaker/implantable cardiac defibrillator.
_____ Rhythm disturbance.
_____ Heart valve disease.
_____ Heart failure.
_____ Heart transplantation.
_____ Congenital heart disease.

Symptoms:
_____ You experience chest discomfort with exertion.
_____ You experience unreasonable breathlessness.
_____ You experience dizziness, fainting, or blackouts.
_____ You take heart medications.
_____ Other health issues.
_____ You have diabetes.
_____ You have asthma or other lung disease.
_____ You have burning or cramping sensation in your legs when walking short
                   distances
_____ You have musculoskeletal problems that limit your physical activity.
_____ You have concerns about the safety of exercise.
_____ You take prescription medication(s).
_____ You are pregnant

Cardiovascular risk factors:
_____ You are a man older than 45 years.
_____ You are a woman older than 55 years, have had a hysterectomy, or are post-
                   menopausal.
_____ You smoke, or quit smoking within the previous 6 months.

_____ Your blood pressure is greater than 140/90 mm Hg (Last date checked:
            _____).
_____ You do not know your blood pressure.
_____ You take blood pressure medication.
_____ Your blood cholesterol level is greater than 200 mg/dl (Last date checked:
            _____).
_____ You do not know your cholesterol level.
_____ You have a close blood relative who had a heart attack or heart surgery
            before age of 55 (father or brother) or age 65 (mother or sister).
_____ You are physically inactive (i.e., you get <30 minutes of physical activity on
            at least 3 days per week).
_____ You are greater than 20 pounds overweight.

Date of Birth: _____

Address: _____
         _____

Email: _____

Physician: _____

REFERENCES

REFERENCES

Abraham, W. M. (1977). Factors in delayed muscle soreness. *Medicine and Science in Sports*, *9*(1), 11-20.

Allen, D. G. (2001). Eccentric muscle damage: mechanisms of early reduction of force. *Acta Physiologica Scandanavica, 171*, 311–319.

Aminian-Far, A., Hadian, M. R., Olyaei, G., Talebian, S., & Bakhtiary, A. H. (2011). Whole-body vibration and the prevention and treatment of delayed-onset muscle soreness. *Journal of Athletic Training, 46*(1), 43-49.

Appell, H. J., Soares, J. M., & Duarte, J. A. (1992). Exercise, muscle damage and fatigue. *Sports Medicine, 13*(2), 108-115.

Armstrong, R. B. (1984). Mechanisms of exercise-induced delayed onset muscular soreness. *Medicine & Science in Sports & Exercise, 16*(6), 529-538.

Baird, M. F., Graham, S. M., Baker, J. S., & Bickerstaff, G. F. (2012). Creatine-kinase- and exercise-related muscle damage implications for muscle performance and recovery. *Journal of Nutrition and Metabolism,* 1-13.

Bajaj, P., Arendt-Nielsen, L., Madeleine, P., & Svensson, P. (2003). Prophylactic tolperisone for post exercise muscle soreness causes reduced isometric force. *European Journal of Pain, 7*(5), 407-418.

Baker, S. J., Kelly, N. M., & Eston, R. G. (1997). Pressure pain tolerance at different sites on the quadricepss femoris prior to and following eccentric exercise. *European Journal of Pain, 1*(3), 229-233.

Bakhtiary, A. H., Safavi-Farokhi, Z., & Aminian-Far, A. (2007). Influence of vibration

on delayed onset of muscle soreness following eccentric exercise. *British Journal

of Sports Medicine, 41*(3), 145-148.

Barnett, A. (2006). Using recovery modalities between training sessions in elite athletes.

Sports Medicine, 36(9), 781-796.

Bobbert, M. F., Hollander, A. P., & Huijing, P. A. (1986). Factors in delayed onset

muscular soreness of man. *Medicine & Science in Sports & Exercise, 18*(1), 75-

81.

Bogaerts, A., Delecluse, C., Claessens, A., Troosters, T., Boonen, S., & Verschueren, S.

(2009). Effects of whole body vibration training on cardiorespiratory fitness and

muscle strength in older individuals (a 1-year randomized controlled trial). *Age

and Aging, 38*(4), 448-454.

Bosco, C., Cardinale, M., Tsarpela, O., & Locatelli, E. (1999). New trends in training

science: the use of vibrations for enhancing performance. *New Study of Athletics,

14*(4), 55–62.

Brand, R. A., Crowninshield, R. D., Wittstock, C. E., Pedersen, D. R., Clark, C. R., &

van Krieken, F. M. (1982). A model of lower extremity muscular anatomy.

Journal of Biomechanical Engineering, 104(4), 304-310.

Broadbent, S., Rousseau, J. J., Thorp, R. M., Choate, S. L., Jackson, F. S., & Rowlands,

D. S. (2010). Vibration therapy reduces plasma IL6 and muscle soreness after

downhill running. *British Journal of Sports Medicine, 44*(12), 888-894.

Brooke-Wavell, K., & Mansfield, N. J. (2009). Risks and benefits of whole body vibration training in older people. *Age and Aging, 38*(3), 254-255.

Brown, D., Chevalier, G., & Hill, M. (2010). Pilot study on the effect of grounding on delayed-onset muscle soreness. *Journal of Alternative and Complementary Medicine, 16*(3), 265-273.

Byrne, C., Twist, C., & Eston, R. (2004). Neuromuscular function after exercise-induced muscle damage: Theoretical and applied implications. *Sports Medicine, 34*(1), 49-69.

Byrnes, W. C., & Clarkson, P. M. (1986). Delayed onset muscle soreness and training. *Clinics in Sports Medicine, 5*(3), 605-614.

Cheung, K., Hume, P., & Maxwell, L. (2003). Delayed onset muscle soreness: Treatment strategies and performance factors. *Sports Medicine, 33*(2), 145-164.

Clarkson, H. (2005). *Joint motion and function assessment.* Philadelphia, PA: Lippincott Williams & Wilkins.

Close, G. L., Ashton, T., McArdle, A., & Maclaren, D. P. (2005). The emerging role of free radicals in delayed onset muscle soreness and contraction-induced muscle injury. *Comparative Biochemistry and Physiology. Part A, Molecular & Integrative Physiology, 142*(3), 257-266.

Coudreuse, J. M., Dupont, P., & Nicol, C. (2004). Delayed post effort muscle soreness. *Annals of Physical and Rehabilitation Medicine, 47*(6), 290-298.

Crameri, R. M., Aagaard, P., Qvortrup, K., Langberg, H., Olesen, J., & Kjaer, M. (2007). Myofibre damage in human skeletal muscle: effects of electrical stimulation versus voluntary contraction. *Journal of Physiology, 583*(1), 365-380.

Dandanell, R., & Engstrom, K. (1986). Vibration from riveting tools in the frequency range 6 Hz-10 MHz and Raynaud's phenomenon. *Scandinavian Journal of Work, Environment & Health, 12*(4), 338-342.

Delecluse, C., Roelants, M., & Verschueren, S. (2003). Strength increase after whole-body vibration compared with resistance training. *Medicine & Science in Sports & Exercise, 35*(6), 1033-1041.

de Weijer, V. C., Gorniak, G. C., & Shamus, E. (2003). The effect of static stretch and warm-up exercise on hamstring length over the course of 24 hours. *Journal of Orthopedic Sports Physical Therapy, 33*(12), 727-733.

Eklund, G., & Hagbarth, K. E. (1966). Normal variability of tonic vibration reflexes in man. *Experimental Neurology, 16*(1), 80-92.

Elmer, S., & Martin J. (2013). Construction of an isokinetic eccentric cycle ergometer for research and training. *Journal of Applied Biomechanics, 29*(4), 490-495.

Elmer, S., McDaniel J., & Martin, J. (2010). Alterations in neuromuscular function and perceptual responses following acute eccentric cycling exercise. *European Journal of Applied Physiology, 110*(6), 1225-1233.

Fagnani, F., Giombini, A., Di Cesare, A., Pigozzi, F., & Di Salvo, V. (2006). The effects of a whole-body vibration program on muscle performance and flexibility in

female athletes. *American Journal of Physical Medicine & Rehabilitation /*
Association of Academic Physiatrists, 85(12), 956-962.

Fielding, R. A., Manfredi, T. J., Ding, W., Fiatarone, M. A., Evans, W. J., & Cannon, J.
G. (1993). Acute phase response in exercise. *American Journal of Physiology,*
265(1), 166-172.

Francis, K. T., & Hoobler, T. (1987). Effects of aspirin on delayed muscle soreness.
Journal of Sports Medicine and Physical Fitness, 27(3), 333-337.

Friden, J., & Lieber, R. L. (1992). Structural and mechanical basis of exercise-induced
muscle injury. *Medicine and Science in Sports and Exercise, 24*(5), 521-530.

Goldspink, G. (1985). Malleability of the motor system: a comparative approach. *Journal*
of Experimental Biology, 115, 375-391

Gormley, S., Swain, D., High, R., Spina, R., Dowling, E., Kotipalli, U., & Gandrakota, R.
(2008). Effect of intensity of aerobic training on VO2max. *Medicine and Science*
in Sports and Exercise, 40(7), 1336-1343.

Gulick, D. T., Kimura, I. F., Sitler, M., Paolone, A., & Kelly, J. D. (1996). Various
treatment techniques on signs and symptoms of delayed onset muscle soreness.
Journal of Athletic Training, 31(2), 145-152.

Hammouda, O., Chahed, H., Chtourou, H., Ferchichi, S., & Miled, A. (2012) Morning-to-
evening difference of biomarkers of muscle injury and antioxidant status in young
trained soccer players. *International Journal of Sports Medicine, 33*(11), 886-891.

Harvey, D. (1998). Assessment of the flexibility of elite athletes using the modified
Thomas test. *British Journal of Sports Medicine, 32*(1), 68-70.

Hasson, S. M., Daniels, J. C., Divine, J. G., Niebuhr, B. R., Richmond, S., Stein, P. G., & Williams, J. H. (1993). Effect of ibuprofen use on muscle soreness, damage, and performance: A preliminary investigation. *Medicine & Science in Sports & Exercise, 25*(1), 9-17.

Herbert, R. D., & Gabriel, M. (2002). Effects of stretching before and after exercising on muscle soreness and risk of injury: Systematic review. *British Medical Journal, 325*(7362), 468.

Hough, T. (1902). Ergographic studies in muscular fatigue and soreness. *American Journal of Physiology, 7*, 76-92.

Imtiyaz, S., Veqar, Z., & Shareef, M. Y. (2014). To compare the effect of vibration therapy and massage in prevention of delayed onset muscle soreness (DOMS). *Journal of Clinical and Diagnostic Research, 8*(1), 133-136.

Issurin, V. B., Liebermann, D. G., & Tenenbaum, G. (1994). Effect of vibratory stimulation training on maximal force and flexibility. *Journal of Sports Sciences, 12*(6), 561-566.

Johnson, B. L., Adamczyk, J. W., Tennoe, K. O., & Stromme, S. B. (1976). A comparison of concentric and eccentric muscle training. *Medicine & Science in Sports & Exercise, 8*, 35–38.

Jonhagen, S., Ackermann, P., & Saartok, T. (2009). Forward lunge: A training study of eccentric exercises of the lower limbs. *Journal of Strength and Conditioning Research, 23*(3), 972-978.

Kanda, K., Sugama, K., Hayashida, H., Sakuma, J., Kawakami, Y., Miura, S., . . . Suzuki, K. (2013). Eccentric exercise-induced delayed-onset muscle soreness and changes in markers of muscle damage and inflammation. *Exercise Immunology Review, 19*, 72-85.

Kosar, A. C., Candow, D. G., & Putland, J. T. (2012). Potential beneficial effects of whole-body vibration for muscle recovery after exercise. *Journal of Strength and Conditioning Research, 26*(10), 2907-2911.

Lau, W. Y., & Nosaka, K. (2011). Effect of vibration treatment on symptoms associated with eccentric exercise-induced muscle damage. *American Journal of Physical Medicine & Rehabilitation, 90*(8), 648-657.

Lecarpentier, Y. (2007). Physiological role of free radicals in skeletal muscles. *The Journal of Applied Physiology, 103*(6), 1917-1918.

Leong, C., McDermott, W., Elmer, S., & Martin, J. (2013). Chronic eccentric cycling improves quadriceps muscle structure and maximum cycling power. *International Journal of Sports Medicine, 35*(7), 559-565.

Luo, J., Mcnamara, B., & Moran, K. (2005). The use of vibration training to enhance muscle strength and power. *Sports Medicine, 35*(1), 23-41.

MacDougall, J., Hicks, A., & MacDonald, J. (1998). Muscle performance and enzymatic adaptations to sprint interval training. *The Journal of Applied Physiology, 10*(3), 571-576.

MacIntyre, D., Reid, W., & McKenzie, D. (1995). Delayed muscle soreness: The inflammatory response to muscle injury and its clinical implications. *Sports Medicine, 41*(6), 392–397.

McDaniel, J., Durstine, J., Hand, G., & Martin, J. (2002). Determinants of metabolic cost during submaximal cycling. *Journal of Applied Physiology, 93*(3) 823-828.

Morgan, D. L., & Proske, U. (2004). Popping sarcomere hypothesis explains stretch-induced muscle damage. *Clinical and Experimental Pharmacology and Physiology, 31*(8), 541-545

Myers, B. A., Jenkins, W. L., Killian, C., & Rundquist, P. (2014). Normative data for hop tests in high school and collegiate basketball and soccer players. *International Journal of Sports Physical Therapy, 9*(5), 596-603.

Peer, K. S., Barkley, J. E., & Knapp, D. M. (2009). The acute effects of local vibration therapy on ankle sprain and hamstring strain injuries. *Physician and Sports Medicine, 37*(4), 31-38.

Pescatello, L. S., & American College of Sports Medicine. (2014). ACSM's guidelines for exercise testing and prescription. 9th edition. *Wolters Kluwer/Lippincott Williams & Wilkins Health.*

Polianskis, R., Graven-Nielsen, T., & Arendt-Nielsen, L. (2001). Computer-controlled pneumatic pressure algometry—a new technique for quantitative sensory testing. *European Journal of Pain, 5*(3), 267-277.

Prisby, R., Lafage-Proust, M., Malaval, L., Belli, A., & Vico, L. (2008). Effects of whole body vibration on the skeleton and other organ systems in man and animal models: What we know and what we need to know. *Aging Research Reviews*, *7*(4), 319-329.

Proske, U., & Morgan, D. (2001). Muscle damage from eccentric exercise: mechanism, mechanical signs, adaptation and clinical applications. *The Journal of Physiology*, *537*, 333-345.

Roelants, M., Verschueren, S., Delecluse, C., Levin, O., & Stijnen, V. (2006). Whole-body-vibration–induced increase in leg muscle activity during different squat exercises. *The Journal of Strength and Conditioning Research*, *20*(1), 124-129.

Schoenfeld, B. (2012). Does exercise-induced muscle damage play a role in skeletal muscle hypertrophy? *The Journal of Strength and Conditioning Research*, *26*(5), 1441-1453.

Schwane, J. A., Johnson, S. R., Vandenakker, C. B., & Armstrong, R. B. (1983). Delayed-onset muscular soreness and plasma CPK and LDH activities after downhill running. *Medicine and Science in Sports and Exercise*, *15*(1), 51-56.

Shinohara, M., Moritz, C. T., Pascoe, M. A., & Enoka, R. M. (2005). Prolonged muscle vibration increases stretch reflex amplitude, motor unit discharge rate, and force fluctuations in a hand muscle. *Journal of Applied Physiology*, *99*(5), 1835-1842.

Siegmund L., Barkley J., Knapp D., & Peer K. (2014). Acute effects of local vibration with biomechanical muscle stimulation on low-back flexibility and perceived stiffness. *Journal of Athletic Training*, *6*(1), 37-45.

Sinert, R., Kohl, L., Rainone, T., & Scalea, T. (1994). Exercise-induced rhabdomyolysis. *Annals of Emergency Medicine*, *23*(6), 1301-1306.

Stauber, W. T. (1989). Eccentric action of muscles: Physiology, injury, and adaptation. *Exercise and Sport Sciences Reviews, 17*, 157-185.

Stay, J. C., Richard, M. D., Draper, D. O., Schulthies, S. S., & Durrant, E. (1998). Pulsed ultrasound fails to diminish delayed-onset muscle soreness symptoms. *Journal of Athletic Training, 33*(4), 341-346.

Tiemessen, I., Hulshof, C., & Frings-Dresen, M. (2008). Low back pain in drivers exposed to whole body vibration: Analysis of a dose-response pattern. *Occupational and Environmental Medicine, 65*(10), 667-675.

Triffletti, P., Litchfield, P. E., Clarkson, P. M., & Byrnes, W. C. (1988). Creatine kinase and muscle soreness after repeated isometric exercise. *Medicine & Science in Sports & Exercise, 20*(3), 242-248.

Veqar, Z. (2014). To compare the effect of vibration therapy and massage in prevention of Delayed Onset Muscle Soreness (DOMS). *Journal of Clinical and Diagnostic Research, 8*(1), 133-136.

Vickers, A. (2001). Time course of muscle soreness following different types of exercise. *BMC Musculoskeletal Disorders, 2*, 5.

Wysocki, A., Butler, M., & Shamliyan, T. (2011). Whole-body vibration therapy for osteoporosis. *Agency for Healthcare Research and Quality. Comparative Effectiveness Technical Briefs*, 10.

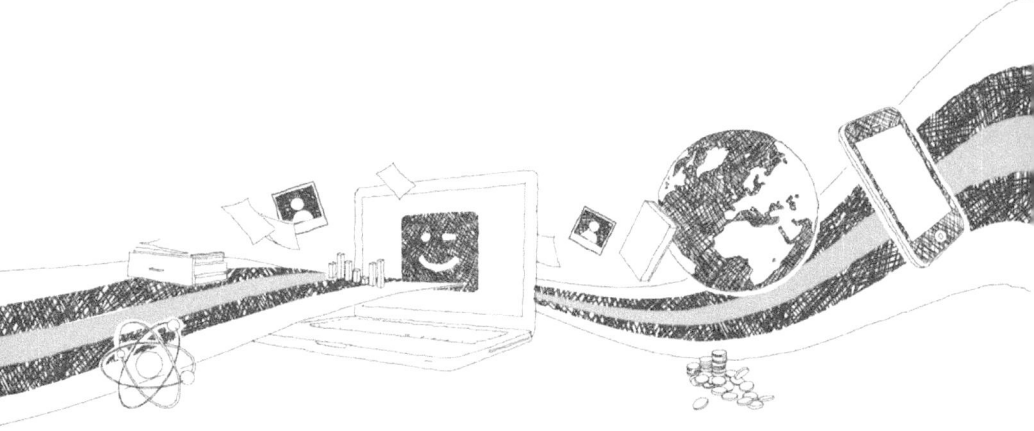
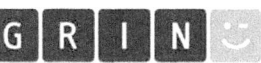